Acknowledgements

HESA would like to express its thanks to the following individuals for their invaluable assistance:

Scott Foley, who designed the book's cover;

Shari Lawler, HESA's Science Editor;

Lisa Whaley Foley, Joy Johnson, and Martha Myers, for formatting assistance;

Dilan Walpola, HESA's creative design consultant;

Nicola Nelson, who wrote the expository text and oversaw editing and preparation of the manuscript;

Susan Foley, who conceived the idea for the book, conducted patient interviews to allow those who were unable to write to be included in the book, and co-edited the manuscript; and

Hinshaw & Culbertson LLP and Yashekia Simpkins, who generously provided legal assistance to enable HESA to become the first nonprofit organization in the world dedicated to Hashimoto's Encephalopathy.

Understanding Hashimoto's Encephalopathy

A Guide for Patients, Families and Caregivers

Featuring Stories of HE Patients from Around the World

By the Hashimoto's Encephalopathy SREAT Alliance
("HESA")

This book is not intended as a substitute for the medical advice of a trained physician. The reader should consult a physician in matters relating to his/her health and particularly with respect to symptoms that may require diagnosis or medical attention. Your physician will use your individual symptoms and health condition to treat you. A book cannot take the place of a trained physician.

Edited by Nicola Nelson and Susan Foley

ISBN-13: 9781484883099
ISBN-10: 1484883098
Library of Congress Control Number: 2013921722
CreateSpace Independent Publishing Platform
North Charleston, South Carolina

Dedication

To the courageous HE/SREAT patients and their loved ones who shared their stories for this book, and to Anji Hogan-Fesler, creator of the first Facebook community for those with HE/SREAT.

Table of Contents

Forward

Hashimoto's Encephalopathy ("HE"), also commonly referred to as Steroid Responsive Encephalopathy Associated with Thyroiditis ("SREAT"), is a rare and devastating autoimmune disease in which a patient's antibodies mistakenly turn on and attack the patient's brain. The results of the attack may include severe cognitive impairment, speech disorders, seizures, memory loss, impaired balance, movement disorders, and sometimes psychosis. Patients sometimes fall into a coma, and in rare cases, die.

Unfortunately, HE is not well understood and patients often face an enormous struggle trying to find the correct diagnosis for their confusing constellation of symptoms. Many neurologists have never even heard of the condition, although that has begun to change in the last few years. Misdiagnosis is the rule more often than the exception, at least in the early months of illness.

HE patients and their families almost universally find themselves having to do their own research in order to try and figure out what to expect, what their treatment options are, and how best to cope. Until now, there has never been a book about HE, and the majority of information about the disease has appeared in scientific journals and isolated case studies which are often difficult if not impossible for patients and their families to access and understand.

This book brings together scientific information, a comprehensive list of resources, and at its core, a collection of narratives by and about HE patients around the world which chronicle their personal experiences, treatments, and outcomes.

The book you hold in your hands is largely the result of an effort by HE patients, families, and caregivers to pool their collective information, experiences, and advice in order to help others better understand this perplexing disease.

But before it became a collective effort, it was originally the brainchild of three women with Hashimoto's Encephalopathy: Anji Hogan-Fesler, Susan Foley, and Nicola Nelson.

Each of these women responded to their diagnosis – when they eventually received it – by trying to learn as much as possible about HE. Each discovered just how hard it is to find information about the disease, and how little support there is for those with HE. And each was determined to do what they could to change that.

Anji formed a Facebook community in which HE patients could find one another and compare notes about treatment, symptoms, and life with HE. Susan recognized the importance and value of the information being shared by the HE patients in Anji's Facebook group, and along with Nicola, determined to collect and archive those stories in a book. Nicola formed the first nonprofit organization in the world devoted to Hashimoto's Encephalopathy, created a website to share HE information and resources, and began investigating the nuts and bolts of publishing a book.

The end result is this book, which was borne of the desire of three women to take the fiery pain of their experience with HE and transform it into a force for good.

In the pages ahead you will learn what HE is, how it is diagnosed – and often misdiagnosed – and how it is treated. You will read stories of courage and heartbreak, of determination and grief, written by mothers, engineers, students, nurses, scientists, and social workers. You will find a variety of HE resources, including lists of support groups, organizations, and internet links with helpful information. In addition, you will find citations to 105 scientific articles about HE published since 2010, so that you can delve as deeply as you like into the science of HE.

HE is unquestionably a powerful and devastating disease, but we – the patients, families, friends and caregivers – believe we are stronger, and we refuse to be defeated.

Welcome to our world. May your journey with us bring you hope, courage, and understanding.

Please note: This book is not intended as a substitute for the medical advice of your physician(s). The reader should always consult a physician in matters relating to his/her health and particularly with respect to symptoms that may require diagnosis or medical attention. Your physician will use your individual symptoms and conditions to treat you. This book cannot take the place of a trained physician.

I. What is Hashimoto's Encephalopathy?

Hashimoto's Encephalopathy ("HE"), also commonly known as Steroid Responsive Encephalopathy Associated with Thyroiditis ("SREAT"), is a rare autoimmune disease characterized by neurological and psychiatric symptoms, and is one of the listed "rare diseases" with the NIH's Genetic and Rare Diseases Information Center.

The generally accepted view is that HE was first described in the medical literature in 1966, when the journal Lancet published an article by British physicians who reported an unusual case involving a 48-year old man who presented with hypothyroidism, multiple episodes of encephalopathy (brain dysfunction, typically characterized by an altered mental state), stroke-like symptoms, and Hashimoto's thyroiditis *[Brain L, Jellinek EH, Ball K: "Hashimoto's Disease and Encephalopathy." Lancet, 1966; 2: 512–514.]*.

It should be noted, however, that a condition called Myxedema psychosis, or myxedema madness, featuring progressive dementia, delirium, and psychosis in those with thyroiditis, was described by Dr. Richard Asher of London in 1949 *[Heinrich TW, Grahm G: "Hypothyroidism Presenting as Psychosis: myxedema madness revisited." Primary Care Companion to the Journal of Clinical Psychiatry, 2003; 5 (6): 260–266.]*.

In the years since the publication of the 1966 article in Lancet, physicians around the globe have continued to observe patients who present with a curious array of neurological and psychiatric symptoms that may include cognitive impairment, seizures, movement disorders, speech disturbances, ataxia, memory loss, headaches, sleep disorders, and psychosis.

Because many of these encephalopathic patients were found to have Hashimoto's Thyroiditis ("HT"), the disorder was originally named Hashimoto's Encephalopathy, to indicate the presence of severe brain dysfunction in those with HT. However many scientists argue that HE is a misnomer, since there appears to be no causal relationship between Hashimoto's Thyroiditis and Hashimoto's Encephalopathy.

In the search for a more appropriate name, scientists have proposed a number of alternative designations, including: Steroid Responsive Encephalopathy Associated with Thyroiditis ("SREAT"), Encephalopathy Associated with Autoimmune Thyroid Disease ("EAATD"), and Non-vasculitic Autoimmune Inflammatory Meningoencephalitis ("NAIM"). Others refer to the disease using the more generic term Autoimmune Encephalopathy ("AE"). Because the scientific community has not yet reached a consensus on the most appropriate name, this book utilizes the abbreviation "HE" to designate the illness, based on the original and still widely-used name.

Although physicians continued to encounter patients with symptoms of HE between 1966 and 1999, few articles or case studies about HE were published during that time period. In fact, many physicians expressed skepticism about the very existence of the enigmatic illness. Some even posited that it was simply a form of conversion disorder.

Beginning in 2000, however, the number of researchers studying HE escalated rapidly, and between 2010 and 2013 over 100 scientific articles and case studies about HE were published by scientists and researchers around the world. A list of many of these journal articles published between 2010 and 2013 appears later in this book.

What causes HE?

Researchers generally agree that HE is caused when the body's immune system becomes confused and begins to attack healthy tissue, but scientists have not yet pinpointed what triggers the autoimmune process to begin. Many patients report first noticing symptoms after an illness or intense period of stress, but this remains purely anecdotal at this point.

Scientists are investigating a variety of possibilities as to the real cause(s) of HE, but no cause has been identified. While a diagnosis of HE requires the presence of antithyroid antibodies in the blood, numerous studies have concluded that HE symptom severity does not correlate to the levels of those antibodies in the blood, and many people have antithyroid antibodies in their blood and do not develop encephalopathy. Because antithyroid antibodies do not appear to cause HE symptoms, researchers are studying other possibilities.

An early theory for the cause of HE is some form of autoimmune inflammation of the blood vessels in the brain or 'autoimmune cerebral vasculitis' *[Forchetti CM, Katsamakis G, Garron DC: "Autoimmune Thyroiditis and a Rapidly Progressive Dementia: global hypoperfusion on SPECT scanning suggests a possible mechanism." Neurology, 1997; 49: 623–626.]*. This theory is still being actively investigated, and finds some support in a variety of articles where SPECT imaging reveals a reduction in blood flow ('hypoperfusion') in the brain during active HE flares, and a resolution of hypoperfusion following steroid treatment *[Kim SJ, Jeung EH, Park MK, Choi S, and Park KW: "Serial Changes in Diffusion-Weighted Magnetic Resonance Images with Hypoperfusion on Brain SPECT in a Case of Hashimoto's Encephalopathy: understanding pathophysiology of Hashimoto's encephalopathy." Dementia and Neurocognitive Disorders, 2013 Mar 31; 12 (1): 29-32.]*. Autoimmune cerebral vasculitis is, therefore, a popular theory for the cause of relapsing-remitting forms of HE.

Alternatively, a 2003 Scottish review suggested that HE is a recurrent form of acute disseminated encephalomyelitis

(ADEM) involving vasculopathy accompanied by blood-brain barrier breakdown *[Chaudhuri A, Behan PO: "The Clinical Spectrum, Diagnosis, Pathogenesis and Treatment of Hashimoto's Encephalopathy (recurrent acute disseminated encephalomyelitis)." Current Medicinal Chemistry, 2003 Oct; 10 (19): 1945-1953.]*. A 2006 recap of the findings suggests this theory is supported by the disease's readily-reversible, rather than destructive, nature (which may represent cerebral edema), the absence of vessel destruction, the low mortality rate, and the frequent near-complete recovery of patients, both clinically and on imaging studies.

A number of studies have explored the possible role of antithyroid antibodies in the cerebrospinal fluid (CSF) of HE patients. Findings vary, but thyroid antibodies in CSF are generally not believed to cause HE symptoms. A 2002 Japanese case study reported that anti-TPO antibodies in an HE patient's CSF disappeared after treatment with steroids *[Saito H, Fujita N, Miyakoshi M, Arai A, Nagai H: "A Case of Hashimoto's Encephalopathy Associated with Graves' Disease." Rinsho Shinkeigaku, 2002 Jul; 42 (7): 619-622.]*. In 2003, Italian researchers reported finding intrathecally-synthesized antithyroid antibodies in the CSF of six HE patients and not in the CSF of 21 controls, but indicated that antibody levels were independent of the patients' clinical status or therapy *[Ferracci F, Moretto G, Candeago RM, Cimini N, Conte F, Gentile M, Papa N, Carnevale A: "Antithyroid Antibodies in the CSF: their role in the pathogenesis of*

Hashimoto's encephalopathy." Neurology, 2003 Feb 25; 60 (4): 712-714.]. In 2004, Japanese researchers published a case study in which antithyroid antibodies in the CSF resolved with steroid therapy, and suggested that the thyroid antibodies were present in the CSF of this HE patient due to a compromised blood-brain barrier *[Wakai M, Nishikage H, Goshima K: "Reversible White Matter Lesions and Antithyroid Antibodies in the Cerebrospinal Fluid in Hashimoto's Encephalopathy: a case report." Rinsho Shinkeigaku, 2004 Jul; 44 (7): 432-437.].*

In recent years, researchers in Japan and other countries have been exploring anti alpha-enolase antibodies as possible biomarkers for HE. Anti-alpha-enolase antibodies occur in association with a variety of infectious and autoimmune illnesses (including HE), and could damage the thin lining of blood and lymphatic vessels, interfere with the dissolving of blood clots, and in some cases induce cell death *[Terrier B, Degand N, Guilpain P, Servettaz A, Guillevin L, Mouthon L: "Alpha-enolase: a target of antibodies in infectious and autoimmune diseases." Autoimmunity Reviews; 6 (2007) 176–182.].* A specific type of anti-alpha-enolase antibody (against the NH2 terminal) is being studied as a potential diagnostic biomarker for HE. Japanese scientists reported in 2013 that these anti-NAE antibodies "are not detected in normal individuals and other disorders such as infections, collagen diseases, multiple sclerosis and other autoimmune conditions. The specificity of the serum anti-NAE Abs is 91% for HE whereas the sensitivity is

50%." *[Kishitani T, Matsunaga A, and Yoneda M: "The Biomarker and Treatment in Hashimoto's Encephalopathy." Japanese Journal of Clinical Medicine, 2013 Jun; 71 (5): 893.].*

It should be noted that it is quite possible for a patient to have more than one type of antibody at a time. For example, in 2010 the Mayo Clinic published a summary across 72 patients with suspected 'autoimmune dementia' (or patients with altered cognition as the principal clinical presentation). These included 40 with anti-TPO antibodies, of which 40% also showed one to three neural autoantibodies out of six tested *[Flanagan EP, McKeon A, Leonnon VA, Boeve BF, Trenerry MR, Tan KM, Drubach DA, Josephs KA, Britton JW, Mandrekar JN, Lowe V, Parisi JE, and Pittock SJ: "Autoimmune Dementia: clinical course and predictors of immunotherapy response." Mayo Clinic Proceedings, 2010 Oct; 85 (10): 881-897.].* As the causal agent (or agents) of HE are not yet known, and the presence of one antibody does not preclude the presence of another, it is possible that antibody diversity may account for some of the variety in HE symptoms and treatment response.

Who gets HE?

Published case studies have included male and female patients of Caucasian, Hispanic, Asian, and African descent, and from all age groups. Patient stories in this book indicate HE can strike people from all walks of life.

A number of researchers have attempted to put some metrics around HE across case reports, but for a variety of reasons it would be difficult to call any of these 'definitive'. Case summaries are generally based on small patient populations, use different criteria for inclusion, and may not include comprehensive demographic or health history details. Tests and findings across case reports often vary widely. There is also suspicion that HE is underdiagnosed, and perhaps not consistently diagnosed across populations. This makes it difficult to give reliable metrics about what the 'typical' HE patient looks like, and thus what we think we know about the face of HE has changed over time, as research advances. Patients, caregivers and physicians may still encounter online claims that one set of findings or statistics represents 'the truth about HE', but are encouraged to view such assertions "with a grain of salt."

A 2004 study published by Italian researchers suggests the prevalence of HE may be 2.1/100,000. Estimates of HE distribution by age and gender vary considerably. HE diagnosis does occur more frequently in women than men, in a ratio that appears to be at least 2:1. Documented diagnoses have occurred in all decades of life, but presently diagnosis appears to be most common in patients in their 40's and 50's. A 2006 literature review indicated approximately 20% of reported cases were in patients younger than 18 years of age, and that clinical findings did not differ by age. It is unclear how closely patterns of diagnosis match patterns of HE occurrence (or in other words, what demographic patterns may exist in HE sufferers who remain undiagnosed or misdiagnosed). In recent years there has been greater awareness and reporting of pediatric HE cases, and the long-term impact on the overall statistical portrait of HE is yet to be seen. The patients whose stories appear in this book range in age from 10 to 65 at the time of diagnosis.

For those who like details, a cross-section of research statistics shows how tough it is to quantify 'who gets HE' – and why readers may want to view with skepticism any single-study HE statistics presented online as absolutes. For example, a 2000 article from Southern Medical Journal summarized statistics across ten reports published between 1974 and 1996, and indicated that "The average age of onset in reported cases is 47 years (range, 14 to 78 years). Approximately 85% of the patients are women." *[Chen, M: "Hashimoto's Encephalopathy." Southern Medical Journal, 2000; 93 (5).]* By contrast, a 2005 article by British researchers states that "Females are more affected than males (3.6:1), with a mean age of onset of 41 years." *[Jacob S, Rajabally YA: "Hashimoto's Encephalopathy: steroid resistance and response to intravenous immunoglobulins." Journal of Neurology, Neurosurgery & Psychiatry, 2005; 76: 455-456.]* Yet a 2006 Mayo Clinic retrospective analysis of 20 patients (female to male ratio 2.3:1) reports a median age at disease onset of 56 years (range of 27 to 84 years). *[Castillo P, Woodruff B, Caselli R, Vernino S, Lucchinetti C, Swanson J, Noseworthy J, Aksamit A, Carter J, Sirven J, Hunder G, Fatourechi V, Mokri B, Drubach D, Pittock S, Lennon V, Boeve B: "Steroid-Responsive Encephalopathy Associated With*

Autoimmune Thyroiditis." Archives of Neurology 2006; 63 (2): 197-202.]. More recently, a 2013 American study reported findings across 13 HE patients, ranging in age from 2 to 66 (median 49). All except one were women (a ratio of 12:1). *[Olmez I, Moses H, Sriram S, Kirshner H, Lagrange AH, Pawate S: "Diagnostic and Therapeutic Aspects of Hashimoto's Encephalopathy." Journal of the Neurological Sciences 2013 Aug 15; (1-2): 67-71.].* The 2010 Mayo Clinic 'autoimmune dementia' analysis included 40 patients with anti-TPO antibodies, of whom 27 were female and 13 were male (a ratio of 2.1:1). Ages at the time of the study (which may differ from the age at symptom onset) ranged 31 to 77, (average 57). *[Flanagan EP, McKeon A, Leonnon VA, Boeve BF, Trenerry MR, Tan KM, Drubach DA, Josephs KA, Britton JW, Mandrekar JN, Lowe V, Parisi JE, and Pittock SJ: "Autoimmune Dementia: clinical course and predictors of immunotherapy response. Mayo Clinic Proceedings, 2010 Oct; 85 (10): 881-897.].*

Little else is currently known about HE risk factors or demographic patterns, but research is expanding rapidly.

What are the symptoms of HE?

This is a difficult question to answer, as HE has so many varied appearances and cases are often reported individually or in small literature reviews, and seldom contain exactly the same tests or conclusions. Patients also very rarely have HE as their only illness, and it can be difficult to isolate whether HE is the actual source of less-common symptoms.

Based on a survey of a variety of analyses characterizing HE, patients typically present with several of the following symptoms – estimates of prevalence vary widely:

- cognitive impairment (including concentration and memory problems)
- emotional, behavioral and personality changes
- speech difficulties (including aphasia or dysphasia)
- tremor
- muscle jerking (myoclonus)
- dizziness, vertigo, and impaired coordination and balance (ataxia)
- headaches
- malaise, weakness, and fatigue
- fluctuating consciousness
- disorientation, confusion, or dementia
- seizures or seizure-like events
- stroke-like episodes
- partial paralysis (often on the right side)
- sleep abnormalities such as insomnia or excessive sleepiness
- sensory or motor difficulties, often on one side
- status epilepticus
- psychosis (including hallucinations, delusions or paranoia)
- coma

HE symptoms are generally reported to follow one of two patterns. In the first type, believed by many researchers to be vasculitic, patients experience a series of relapsing-remitting stroke-like episodes, with transient focal neurological deficits. Symptoms vary in intensity and duration, and can come and go quickly. The second type of HE is progressive, rather than relapsing and remitting. It may be more frequently characterized by dementia and psychiatric symptoms. Many patients, however, display an overlap in symptoms between the two types.

What diagnostic tests are usually done?

HE is a diagnosis of exclusion, and some of the many diagnoses that must be ruled out include toxic, infectious, or metabolic causes, paraneoplastic encephalitis, other autoimmune encephalopathies with known antibodies such as anti-NMDA encephalitis, epilepsy, complications of Hashimoto's thyroiditis or certain types of migraines, and a wide variety of other conditions. Testing will generally include numerous blood tests including antithyroid antibodies, and may include a spinal tap to examine cerebrospinal fluid, an EEG, neurological and neuropsychiatric testing, and / or medical imaging such as CT scan, MRI, PET, or SPECT scan.

What test results are typical of HE?

No single test can confirm a diagnosis of HE and, apart from a negative antithyroid antibody test, no single test result can rule out HE. Diagnosis requires careful consideration of many factors and significant physician discretion. Often diagnosis is a matter of clinical symptoms suggesting encephalopathy, in the presence of a positive antithyroid antibody test and negative test results for other possible causes. Even as researchers are beginning to recognize subtler presentations of HE, timing is still of the essence because delays in treatment increase the risk of permanent neurological damage, coma, and even death.

Science has not yet unlocked all the mysteries of HE, and because there is not yet a definitive lab test to confirm the diagnosis, it remains a diagnosis of exclusion, requiring physicians to run many tests to rule out the other possible causes for patient symptoms before making a diagnosis of HE. Given the high risk of untreated autoimmune encephalopathy, the lack of definitive diagnostic criteria or tests, and the extent of overlap of HE symptoms with other illnesses, some researchers recommend using a trial of corticosteroids or immunotherapy to confirm diagnosis, rather than waiting until diagnosis is confirmed. In a 2013 article, Segers et al suggest "a pragmatic approach involving a short empirical therapeutic trial with intravenous or oral corticoids; this should be considered in all patients with sub acute encephalopathy and with laboratory arguments for an underlying autoimmune aetiology" *[Segers K, Braconnier P, Corazza F, Divano L, Mabrouk A, Robberecht J, and Surquin M: "Subacute Cognitive Deterioration with High Serum Anti-thyroid Peroxidase Antibodies: two cases and a plea for pragmatism." Psychogeriatrics, 2013 Sep 17; 13 (3): 175-179.]*

A 2011 literature review looked at 130 patients across 52 studies *[de Holanda NCP, de Lima DD, Cavalcanti TB, Lucena, and Bandeira F: "Hashimoto's Encephalopathy: systematic review of the literature and an additional case." The Journal of Neuropsychiatry & Clinical Neurosciences, 2011 Sep 1; 23 (4): 384-390.]*. Key findings from this and selected other large studies are summarized below, bearing in mind that some of the less common findings may turn out to be incidental and unrelated to HE.

Antithyroid Antibodies

While symptoms and most lab findings vary by study, one thing remains consistent: by definition, for a diagnosis of HE a patient must have elevated antithyroid antibodies – including anti-thyroid peroxidase antibodies (anti-TPO – formerly called thyroid microsomal antibodies), and / or thyroglobulin antibodies. (It is unclear what role if any may be played by thyrotropin receptor antibodies (TRAbs – also known as TSH receptor or 'TSHR' antibodies), or more recently discovered antithyroid antibodies such as Anti-Na^+/I^- symporter antibodies, megalin (gp330), or pendrin autoantibodies.) The finding of elevated antibodies is 'necessary but not sufficient' to establish an HE diagnosis; the finding of antithyroid antibodies does not mandate a diagnosis of HE, nor does it rule out the presence of any other possible conditions. As long as antithyroid antibody levels are above normal, the actual extent of antibody elevation is not diagnostically significant for HE; numerous studies have established that antithyroid antibody levels do not correlate with severity of encephalopathy symptoms. As with other autoimmune antibodies, antithyroid antibody levels often decrease following steroid therapy, but this is not considered to be clinically significant to the HE diagnosis. Although testing for elevated antibodies is usually based on serum (blood), these elevated antibody levels may be present in CSF (cerebrospinal fluid) as well.

TSH Levels

Patients' TSH levels may be high, normal, or low at time of diagnosis, and patients with Graves' disease are not immune to HE. As long as antithyroid antibodies are present, TSH is only diagnostically relevant to HE if a patient is so severely hypothyroid that it could provide an alternate explanation for the patient's symptoms. Thyroid replacement hormone may be initiated or adjusted to regulate the patient's thyroid levels, but this is not considered a treatment for HE.

EEG

The electroencephalogram studies of HE patients are abnormal in up to 90% of cases, but they are usually nonspecific. A normal EEG does not rule out HE. The most common abnormal findings are diffuse or generalized slowing, and the degree of slowness of the waves is generally related to the clinical severity of the encephalopathy. Other findings may include frontal intermittent rhythmic delta activity (FIRDA), delta and theta activity, triphasic waves, focal and intermittent slowing, epileptiform abnormalities, or photoparoxysmal and photomyogenic responses. Steroid therapy is generally associated with improvement or resolution of EEG abnormalities within weeks.

Cerebrospinal Fluid

Elevated protein levels in cerebrospinal fluid (CSF) are common findings. Oglioclonal bands are occasionally seen. Antithyroid antibodies in CSF are rarely tested for, but are surprisingly common findings that do not confirm or rule out an HE diagnosis.

Medical Imaging

MRIs and CT scans are frequently normal, or contain nonspecific abnormalities regarded as 'within normal limits' based on patient age. MRI scans are the most frequently administered imaging test, and the most common abnormalities detected include hyper-signal on T2 (consistent with edema or brain inflammation), with lesser incidence of findings such as cerebral atrophy and ischemia. CT scans are administered far less often, and common abnormalities detected include cerebral atrophy, ischemic abnormalities and / or cerebral edema. PET and SPECT scans often show reduced blood flow (hypoperfusion). In rare instances, cerebral angiography is performed to check for vasculitis, and is typically normal. Follow-up imaging studies may show improvement after successful treatment, particularly SPECT scans.

Neurological Testing

Depending on the areas of the brain impacted, patients may exhibit a variety of neurological signs. Brisk knee reflexes do not appear to be a focal point in the literature but anecdotally appear to be common and potentially diagnostically useful in corroborating encephalopathy. Given the frequency with which patients anecdotally report symptoms consistent with frontal lobe dysfunction, neurological testing should include screening for frontal lobe dysfunction in addition to other standard neurological tests.

Neuropsychiatric Testing

Patients frequently anecdotally report deterioration of memory, concentration, and processing speed during active

HE flares, with improvement on successful therapy. A 2012 Italian case study reported neuropsychiatric findings before, during, and after successful treatment of HE, and indicated that the subject's residual difficulties evolved toward a selective deficit in executive functions. Anecdotal reports from patients suggest this is not atypical, and even after successful therapy many patients report residual issues typical of frontal lobe dysfunction.

What might HE be mistaken for?

Symptoms of HE overlap with many other conditions, and as the patient stories throughout this book make clear, it is rare for an HE patient to be correctly diagnosed from the onset of symptoms. Instead, most patients receive a variety of misdiagnoses before they are eventually determined to have HE, if in fact they are lucky enough to be correctly diagnosed at all.

Reported case studies indicate patients have been initially misdiagnosed with viral encephalitis, Creutzfeldt-Jakob disease, stroke or transient ischemic attack, psychosis, delirium, depression, bipolar disorder, chronic meningitis, Alzheimer disease, migraine, Lewy body dementia, metabolic encephalopathy, drug-resistant epilepsy, and progressive myoclonus epilepsy syndrome to name just a few. In addition, patients have anecdotally reported being initially diagnosed with conversion disorder, movement disorders, mood disorders, complicated migraine, 'stress', 'the natural process of aging', and being told 'it's all in their head'. With growing awareness of HE, recent case studies also report other illnesses may initially be misdiagnosed as HE, such as anti-NMDAR encephalitis.

How is HE treated?

Initial Intervention

Antiseizure drugs are generally initiated for patients experiencing seizures. Thyroid replacement therapy is often initiated for patients who show subacute or acute hypothyroidism, though this does not correlate with neurological improvement.

The first-line treatment for HE is generally steroids because up to 90% of HE patients respond to steroid treatment. For those severely affected patients who have been hospitalized, treatment is often initiated with a course of high dose IV methylprednisolone, at rates of 1 gr (1000 mg) per day for 3-7 days. Symptoms in some patients may begin to alleviate within as little as 1-2 days after initiating treatment, although improvement is more commonly seen on or after day 3-4. Patients receiving such treatment often return home on a high dose of oral prednisone such as 60 mg/day, and slowly taper down over a 6-12 month period. Alternately, some patients are treated with high doses of IV dexamethasone, or oral prednisone.

For patients who do not respond to steroid therapy, plasma exchange (plasmapheresis) or intravenous immunoglobulins may be considered.

Case studies have been published describing cases of HE that did not respond to steroids, plasmapheresis, or IVIG but improved after total thyroidectomy. Given that thyroid antibodies are not viewed as causative in HE, and that other factors can cause HE to go into remission, it seems risky to assume a reliable cause-and-effect link between thyroidectomy and HE remission. Thyroidectomy case reports also generally do not incorporate an extended period of follow-up observation to monitor for relapse, and internet blogs and online support sites tell the stories of many thyroidectomy patients for whom the surgery appeared to do more harm than good.

Long-term Therapy

Many patients remain on a low-dose of steroids indefinitely in order to keep symptoms to a minimum. Patients who do not respond adequately to initial therapies or who experience multiple relapses may be placed on other long-term immunomodulatory therapies, such as azathioprine, cyclophosphamide, plaquenil, mycophenolate mofetil (CellCept), chloroquine, or methotrexate, and may be given periodic IVIG infusions or plasma exchange.

Spontaneous Remission

Numerous reports of 'spontaneous remission' appear throughout the literature. A 2003 literature review suggested that 17% of cases of HE resolved with thyroid replacement therapy alone, acknowledging that these cases might have been destined to resolve spontaneously. However, case studies that include long-term follow-up report a high incidence of recurrence, consistent with the fluctuation patterns of a relapsing remitting autoimmune disease rather than a spontaneous 'cure.'

Relapses

Where it is reported at all, follow-up time varies across case studies. A 2011 literature review reported that approximately one-quarter of patients relapsed on withdrawal of the corticosteroid, requiring a change in steroid tapering, and 15% relapsed requiring further treatment. Only 8% of the patients studied showed complete remission of symptoms, laboratory, and radiographic changes, and were stable without relapse during the entire follow-up period.

Supplemental Treatments

Patients may also be placed on medications to control specific HE symptoms – such as anticonvulsants, sleep aids, anti-anxiety medications, and memory drugs.

Severe cases of HE may require rehabilitative therapies such as physical, occupational, speech, and cognitive rehabilitation therapy.

Long-term Prognosis

Long-term prognosis for most patients is good, but depends on the severity and type of HE, and the demands of the patient's lifestyle. Those with relapsing remitting HE or significant residual deficits may be unable to maintain their careers, particularly those whose professions require consistent performance, good communication skills, strong memory, and the ability to concentrate. Seizures pose serious risks for some patients, and pediatric HE patients may be at higher risk of developing status epilepticus (uncontrollable seizures). Balance and concentration problems can also create safety issues via increased risk of accidents or falls.

Are any there any complementary treatments that might be helpful?

There is no substitute for formal medical intervention in HE, but in a context of appropriate medical management, patients may also find benefit in supplemental therapies or lifestyle changes.

Even with successful immunotherapy, published case reports indicate many patients have residual symptoms such as forgetfulness, irritability, concentration difficulties, tremor, gait ataxia, and other symptoms. Anecdotal reports from patients suggest a higher degree of residual issues and long-term impairment than appears to be recorded in the literature. Rehabilitation therapies such as cognitive rehabilitation therapy may assist patients in their recovery, and in developing compensating strategies for residual deficits.

A 2008 study from investigators at Harvard teaching hospitals indicates that the 'relaxation response' can immediately alter gene expression for over 2,000 genes, including many tied to inflammation, immune function, metabolism, insulin secretion, and the body's response to stress. While the effect of the relaxation response has not explicitly been studied in relation to HE, evoking the relaxation response may prove to be both enjoyable and beneficial. Practices known to evoke the relaxation response include meditation, repetitive prayer, yoga, tai chi, breathing exercise, progressive muscle relaxation, biofeedback, guided imagery and Qi Gong *[Dusek JA, Otu HH, Wohlhueter AL, Bhasin M, Zerbini LF, et al.: "Genomic Counter-Stress Changes Induced by the Relaxation Response." PLoSONE 2008; 3 (7): e2576.]*.

When dealing with a rare illness, it is important not to overlook the more mundane basics of health. Patients anecdotally report that, consistent with other autoimmune illnesses, germ exposure can cause a 'flare' of symptoms, as can stress and over-exertion. Particularly for those with the relapsing-remitting form of HE, it may help to take extra care to avoid germ exposure. This could be as simple as frequent hand washing and avoiding close contact with people who are sick, or could include steps such as wearing disposable gloves when cleaning a toilet or handling raw meat, or using a dust mask and/or sinus rinse for long-distance air travel. Managing stress, and getting adequate rest and nutrition are likely to remain important to wellness.

As all patients with HE have antithyroid antibodies, it is important to manage any related hypothyroidism carefully. In 2012 the American Association of Clinical Endocrinologists and the American Thyroid Association published clinical practice guidelines for hypothyroidism in adults indicating treatment should be considered for patients whose TSH levels fall in the 'subclinical hypothyroid' range if the patient has symptoms of hypothyroidism, positive TPO antibodies, evidence of cardiovascular disease, or risk factors for cardiovascular disease.

Anecdotally, many HE patients have reported deficiencies in B and D vitamins, which could exacerbate symptoms although the deficiencies may not necessarily have been caused by HE. It may be worthwhile for HE patients to have vitamin levels tested periodically, and to be screened for common MTHFR gene variants that might cause trouble utilizing B vitamins. Some patients also report experiencing benefit from acupuncture or a gluten free diet.

Online HE support groups can be great places for asking what others have found helpful in addressing specific symptoms or side effects, but only a physician can tell an HE patient whether a particular therapy, vitamin, herb, or medication would be advisable in that patient's situation.

Can HE be cured?

Like most autoimmune diseases, at present HE can be treated and can even go into extended remission, but there is no known permanent cure.

Can damage due to HE be 'fixed'?

A number of studies have reported that EEG and imaging abnormalities improved or resolved in response to response to steroid therapy, suggesting that some of the disruption caused by HE may be reversible. However, many patients do report residual deficits. In some cases it is unclear whether the deficits are due to incomplete management of HE (and would be reversible with additional therapy), or whether they represent some sort of more durable damage.

Even in instances of more durable damage, recent research demonstrates that the neuroplasticity of the brain is greater than originally believed. In such instances, cognitive rehabilitation therapy may assist patients in regaining lost abilities, as well as adapting to their 'new normal'.

Is there promising new research for HE?

Research published by Northwestern University in 2012 demonstrated that bits of myelin attached to biodegradable nanoparticles could be used to retrain the immune system and halt a model of relapsing remitting multiple sclerosis (MS) in mice. The nanoparticle was made from an easily produced and already FDA-approved substance, and limited human trials have shown promising results. In 2013, new research indicated that antigen-decorated microparticles could induce long-term T-cell tolerance in mice with relapsing experimental autoimmune encephalomyelitis *[Getts DR, Aaron J Martin AJ, McCarthy DP, Terry RL, Hunter ZN, Yap WT, Getts MT, Pleiss M, Luo X, King NJC, Shea LD, and Miller SD: "Microparticles Bearing Encephalitogenic Peptides Induce T-cell Tolerance and Ameliorate Experimental Autoimmune Encephalomyelitis." Nature Biotechnology, 2012; 30: 1217–1224.]*. This avenue of research appears to hold promise to generate extended remission or even 'cure' for many autoimmune diseases, including HE. For this method to be viable in treating HE, the exact antigen under attack by HE would need to be identified.

Time will tell whether a connection will emerge between anti-NAE antibodies against the NH2 terminal and the autoimmune cerebral vasculitis often theorized to cause relapsing remitting HE, and whether the enolase 1, (alpha) gene that encodes alpha-enolase will contain clues on the development and management of HE.

What can be done in the meantime?

Patients, caregivers and physicians can help raise awareness of HE so that it is considered early in a patient's diagnostic journey, and so that HE organizations are better able to attract research funds to pursue new methods of diagnosis and treatment.

Where can I go for more information?

The foregoing text simply provides an overview of some of the available findings regarding HE. The patient stories at the heart of this book will give a real-world glimpse of what HE looks like through the eyes of 48 HE patients and caregivers, with detailed descriptions of symptoms, tests, and treatments.

The final section of this book, titled "Resources" includes an extensive list of scientific articles which can be used to study in detail the most recent research, case studies, and findings regarding HE. It also includes information on how to connect with a variety of HE support groups.

II. In Our Own Words: Patient Stories

In late 2012 a call went out to the members of the Facebook HE/SREAT community, the Topica Helps online community, the Encephalitis Global online community (via Inspire.com) and HE/SREAT patients generally via several internet blogs, requesting narrative accounts from those who had been officially diagnosed with HE and were willing to share their stories with the world.

What follows are stories that describe the experiences of HE/SREAT patients from the United States, Denmark, Australia, Scotland, and England. Some are short, some are long. Some are detailed, and some are more general. Some are purely descriptive, while others are more reflective in nature. Each is a portrait of a life changed forever by HE.

Through these stories you will meet a variety of people from all walks of life. Wherever possible we have included the patient's age at time of diagnosis, although this information was unavailable in a few instances.

Virtually all of the narratives were written by the patients themselves, and their stories are told in their own words. In a few cases, narratives were written by Susan Foley based on personal interviews she conducted with patients unable to write for themselves, which were then reviewed and authorized by the patients. One story was written by a family member whose loved one succumbed to the sequelae of HE, and two were written by spouses of HE patients too impaired to create their own written accounts. Most patients had to rely on information from family and friends to describe the most severe points in their illness, due to memory loss. In a subsequent chapter, we separately present the story of children with HE, written by their parents.

It is HESA's hope that these stories will help patients, families, caregivers, and clinicians better understand Hashimoto's Encephalopathy.

We begin with the stories of the three women introduced in the Forward, Anji, Susan and Nicola, whose experience with HE ultimately led to the creation of this book.

Anji

I will begin with a brief description of who I am or was. My name is Anji; a very extroverted, social butterfly who loves people, a born helper, a school social worker for 13 years. I met the most wonderful man in 1999 and we married in 2002. We had our first (and only) child, Zakk, in 2003. I was living what I thought to be the perfect life. Then BAM! Out of nowhere I became sick.

It was September 2004 when my first episode reared its ugly head. For a few weeks I had been noticing that my hair was everywhere and falling out in clumps. I thought it was probably a result of pregnancy hormones, since I just had a baby in December 2003. I called my gynecologist and inquired what to do to help stop my hair from falling out.

She explained that the hair loss would be normal IF I was pregnant, but because I had already had Zakk the hormones were not the cause. She gave me the name and number of a neurologist.

On September 28, 2004, I was in my office at school. One of my long-time students had come in to visit. I realized I recognized her, but somehow I could not recall her name nor did I know how I knew her. I had worked with this student for years on grief issues yet on this date I could not recall her name. I made an excuse, telling her I didn't feel well and had to go home.

I then left school and drove home. I called a neurologist on the way and scheduled an appointment. That night I was feeling like myself and kept a dinner/concert date with my husband, Chad. We went downtown with family, for dinner and a concert. We had an Italian dinner at a quaint little restaurant and I had chicken fettuccini, which we would later blame for the night's events.

At the concert, I asked Chad if the music was normally this loud as I was in excruciating pain from the volume of the concert. I left him to enjoy the music and excused myself to the restroom, where I remained there for the duration of the show. I began throwing up and continued to hide there, to shelter myself from the noise of the music. At the end of the concert we all discussed my ailment and the possible cause. We all blamed the chicken and thought I had food poisoning. Little did any of us know the real outcome was much more devastating and deadly.

Once at home I continued to throw up but now had a severe headache, as if a butcher cleaver was chopping through my skull. I cried and screamed, as this was not like any headache I had ever experienced. Chad fed me Advil and gave me a cold compress for my head. We still blamed it all on the chicken.

Right…

On October 2, I noticed a Pottery Barn Halloween Spider bag which I had wanted to get Zakk but hadn't yet bought. It was lying in my living room, with Zakk's name embroidered on it. I picked it up and asked my husband where it had come from. Chad replied that Kristine (my sister-in-law) had bought it a few weeks ago. I thought Chad was fooling around with me. I had completely lost that memory.

The headaches continued. These were not just your typical headaches. They were severe from the onset, causing me to vomit throughout the day and night. Chad called the doctor to get me in to see a neurologist. He was told that if my condition worsened he should take me to the ER.

One night, having never before felt the pain I was experiencing, yelling and writhing in pain, Chad took me to the ER closest to home. I looked like a walking zombie and acted like one. At the hospital I was asked who our president was, what year it was, what my social security number was, and why I was there. I felt very confused and my head was killing me. Finally, relief came. They gave me a morphine shot and it was as if a veil was lifted and the pain was gone. I see why there are drug addicts! I was given a CT scan which showed nothing out of the norm.

Within the next two days we went to an appointment with a neurologist. When we saw Dr. Speal she completed the series of questions which had been presented days earlier. After assessing my condition she said we needed to immediately go to the ER at St. Luke Hospital to be checked in to the hospital. We did as directed.

We drove to my mother's place to pick her up as Chad needed the help and support. On the way to the hospital I attempted to exit the moving car because I felt as if I was being abducted. My mother had to hold me down to prevent my escape. I was acting like a wild animal! Claws, teeth, growling...

At the ER they did a spinal tap (several attempts, I wouldn't hold still, OUCH!) and they found cause to admit me to the hospital immediately: high levels of protein in my spinal fluid and a state of dementia!

During my three month stay at the hospital I underwent many tests, observations and incorrect diagnoses. I forgot everything and everyone in my life but my son. My previously healthy brain (I never got sick and was always healthy as a horse) was now the cause of my demise. I was being attacked by the very thing that helps keep me well: my own antibodies.

They ran the full gamut of tests at the hospital and terms were loosely tossed around: West Nile Virus, poison, Bird Flu, Mad Cow. My mother, frustrated, actually fired the original neurologist and requested the chief neurologist, Dr. Mike Newmark, take on my case. He, along with Dr. Chris Wey (a young, pharmaceutical genius) conducted more tests. Dr. Wey thought I had MS. A brain biopsy (they're gonna cut into what????) was ordered and conducted. I asked the brain surgeon ahead of time if he would perform the same on his wife, since they were proposing to pop my skull off and cut into my brain like in a horror movie. His word comforted me as he said yes, he would allow the same surgery for his wife. The results were negative, but left a permanent reminder as they took a chunk out of the skull! Try hiding that pretty li'l scar.

Dr. Newmark (MY HERO!!) suggested they try chemotherapy, as this would suppress my antibodies (which were elevated). They ordered the treatment and after it was administered I came out of the fog of dementia. I woke up asking what was going on and why I was there. My mother called Chad, who had gone home to spend some time with our son. When he answered the phone she told him, "There is someone here who would like to talk to you."

She handed me the phone and I heard my husband break down and cry when I said, "Hi Chad." He was crying because it had been months since I had been able to communicate with him.

The effects of the chemo lasted only one day, and then I was once again unable to speak or communicate. (I just need a dang break already!)

I was given IV steroids. I also underwent plasmapheresis (plasma exchange) where my plasma was taken out and exchanged for synthetic plasma. Out with the junk plasma and in with the clean. Bye-bye sick antibodies, in with synthetic clean antibodies. To do this they had to surgically insert a tube into my chest (almost to my heart).

Well after weeks of not having a real shower, I just HAD to have one even though I wasn't supposed to. So I took a shower, as I was sick of sponge baths. I inadvertently got the port wet and as a result, it became infected, causing me to relapse. UGH. I underwent a second surgery to insert a new, second port into the opposite side of my cavity. This is when I lost my hearing.

I asked those in my room why the TV was turned down so low. It became clear that I couldn't hear. Audiology tests revealed that I had become 100% deaf in my left ear and more than 50% deaf in my right ear as a result of the antibiotic given to fight the first infection. Seriously, can't I get a break??? Nope.

I underwent plasma exchange for two months: The first week was every day, the next two weeks was every other day, and then we began to go once a week. After the treatments I was very groggy and weak. Once these treatments ceased, I was CellCept, a drug given to transplant patients so their bodies won't reject a new organ. It worked.

During my months living with an unknown condition my eight month old son had lived with his paternal grandparents and Chad stayed by my side. He did not go to work and was my constant strength. Our son, Zakk, had his first birthday in my hospital bed, with Elmo, cake, and our small family. Not the huge event I had imagined. The first birthday is supposed to be a special moment to celebrate your child's life and the parents' survival of the first year, child unscathed. Right. Didn't happen like a Hallmark movie. More like the movie Girl Interrupted.

While in the hospital I thought of escaping many times just to go see and be with Zakk. I was under the impression I was in prison. I even plotted different escape plans but invariably ended up downstairs at the McDonald's in the hospital. I would collect all Chad's loose change to buy hot fudge sundaes. (Have you tried hospital food?) Once my mother told me the McDonald's was closed on Sundays. Umm...no. I had lost memories but not my entire mind! Kinda like the time I was certain that my hair dresser was coming to cut/wash/style my hair in my hospital room. Chad said that the hair place was closed on the weekends but I knew better. I had always had my hair done on a weekend.

Chad did his best, bringing his sickly wife magazines, cross word puzzles and catalogs. He was trying to keep me from going out of my mind (no pun intended). Ha! I used my Pottery Barn customer ID number from the back of a catalog and did a ton of shopping one week: dining room table, rugs, chandeliers. You name it, I bought it, and it was all delivered to my home. Poor Chad had to send all these items back. Try explaining your wife was out of her mind and didn't know what she was doing.

My doctors couldn't explain why I contracted HE. Their best guess was that the pregnancy hormones may have had something to do with it. Because I would never terminate a pregnancy, and my husband didn't me to go through a hysterectomy, he opted to have a vasectomy. This was very difficult for me as I love babies and wanted another. But to ensure our one child would be able to keep his mother (since the doctors told us that the next time I might die) I agreed.

Once I was home, as I began to mend, Chad helped me to re-learn how to drive a car. My mother was not happy about it but Chad was my husband and what he said went. I practiced first by pushing a shopping cart around the store and attempting not to run into things, including people. That was funny, actually. I had lost all memory of the rules of driving. I tried driving to my neighbor's house and then to the grocery store (all against the wishes of others). Then I tried taking quick drives to the mailbox. The biggie was when I tried driving to my neurology appointments ALONE.

I'm so much better now, but I have ongoing impairments, in part because of the many lesions in my brain (yea, a valid excuse!). I have very poor memory retention. I have insomnia too, and my neuro was afraid to give me a narcotic to assist with sleep so I began drinking too much in order to sleep. When I became worried about possible damage to my liver, kidneys and general health I went to a PCP who did not know me or my HE condition and he prescribed Lunesta, which helps.

Today it is very difficult for me to remember names of people. I'm HORRIBLE with simple math (poor Zakk). I get dates and times mixed up, and as a result of the high dosage steroids given to me in the hospital I now have 2 artificial hips. The blood wasn't getting to the needed areas, the veins died, and my hips, which needed that blood supply, didn't receive it. I ended up rubbing bone on bone.

Nevertheless, I have been able to return to being a full-time wife, which I love more than air, and all-the-time mother to a Bipolar, AD/HD, full of life Oppositional Defiant child. I also work as a school social worker and deal with the emotional issues of many students. At one point I began working on a graduate degree, but stopped to be a better mother. I attended real estate school and passed the RE exam, then held a part time job as a licensed Realtor for a year but I allowed my license to lapse because the part time job was more work than my full time job. I held a position in my Home Owners Association as a board member for two years. I continue to work hard to try and prove that I am stronger than HE.

I eat a healthy diet, work out at the gym more days than not, and I love my family more than myself. Someone close to me once asked, after hearing me blame something on my brain damage, "how long can you use that excuse?" My answer? How about for the rest of my life.

This story was very difficult for me to write and I have left out a lot. It's been hard for my husband to relive these horrible memories as he helped me reconstruct events of which I have no memory. All I can say is, ask him what it has been like to live through the HE experience. He lived it too. He is the epitome of what love embodies and I write this story through his loving eyes. Always my calm during my storm.

I want to add a special message to and about my son. I love you, my Zakk. Those big, blue eyes looking up at me make everything all better. You are my strength.

And I want to add that my mother, who wants to save everyone, poured her entire self into helping me get the best medical help. She took the reins when Chad needed help. It was the mother's love that shone through those troubling times. And my in-laws, Roy and Pat Fesler, cared for Zakk when I was ill, and kept our family strong. I can never thank them enough.

In a way, what you just read is my HE story. But for me, there is also a much larger story: the story of how my HE ultimately changed things for people around the world.

The Creation of the Facebook HE Community

When I first I heard the term Hashimoto's Encephalopathy I found myself thinking: "HUH? What? I am so lost! What the heck is Hashimoto's Encephalopathy? It's very rare? Great. Why ME? Now what? There is nothing out there on the internet that I can go to for HE support!

That was when I decided that the best tool for my HE journey and recovery was to come up with my own support system, besides my family, to help me deal with this rare disease.

Social Media was at my fingertips and I was already an avid user of Facebook, so I typed in the key terms, HE, and found nothing was set up. I had no clue how to create a Facebook group, did not know the terms, or if there were any rules that went along with Facebook groups. But I went ahead and started a group for HE and have been learning as I – and we - go. I never expected the Facebook HE group to gain much press or even many members, as I was under the impression that HE was so rare. Now we have over 300 members and we continue to grow.

My goal is to help people find information and support. I am not the wisest, nor do I have all the answers, but as a collective group the members of the Facebook HE community help others along the HE path. Now there is a nonprofit organization dedicated to shedding light on HE, and HE even has its own awareness ribbons, awareness bracelets, a cook book and now this book.

The HE survivors who shared their stories for this book are the faces of HE and we are strong. We are a chosen few, and we hope to encourage and educate many.

Susan

My name is Susan Foley and my story is long. It involves a lot of misdiagnosis, and eventually the right diagnosis: Hashimoto's Encephalopathy/Encephalitis.

Around the year 2005 I started to have some strange symptoms that I tried to ignore. I never got sick, so I thought I could will it all away. Finally as I sat in the parking lot of WalMart one day, looking at the space between my truck and the store, I thought I cannot do it. I do not have the energy to walk from here to there.

But it was Christmas, so I had to force myself through and go. I pushed myself through the store thinking I would never make it. That is when I decided maybe I could no longer ignore how I felt. So I went to see a doctor who diagnosed me with severe hypothyroidism and borderline hypertension. I had been gaining weight, had sore fingers, and could not bend my thumbs without severe pain. I blamed this all on the hypothyroid problems he had diagnosed me with. I bought books to read on the subject, went on thyroid meds, and thought, ok, I will be better soon. Not to be so.

Soon my hair started to dry out - it looked like straw - and I lost all hair on my arms, hands, legs, underarms and in my female private area. I no longer sweated. Again I blamed it on the thyroid problem. I started to feel exhausted, began getting rashes on my face and my arms, and legs. My eyelids itched so badly. My primary physician diagnosed this as photosensitivity, telling me to stay out of the sun and then I'd be fine. Again, not so.

I then got a rash that went from the back side of my legs from my feet to my butt. Then it was on my arms and chest, and it itched intensely. I thought I would not be able to stand it. I could not sleep at night. Doctors tried steroids but as soon as I stopped taking them the rash came back. This lasted from October through March of 2006. It was winter, so this couldn't be blamed on the sun. Then my hands started to get bad. My fingers were swollen, blotched, itched, and would get plaques on them. People would actually stop me and ask me what was wrong with them. I dropped everything I held.

I developed red hot flushes on my arms, and on the inside of my legs from ankles to knees that stayed red for weeks at a time.

I decided to go see a dermatologist, who did every test in the book. I had vials and vials of blood taken checking for things I had never heard of before. He said he was sure it was lupus but did not want to diagnose it as such because I would never be able to get insurance again. So he recorded it as photosensitivity.

At this time my arms became terribly weak and I could not lift them above my head, or hang on to the steering wheel. My legs were weak. I had a hard time walking up a sidewalk curb. I also started to have nonstop diarrhea. Then I had an episode at work that landed me in the ER.

I was working and had a weird sense of not being able to talk. I could not get the words out of my mouth. I felt dizzy and just plain weird. Because of a very serious heart history in my family I agreed to make an ER visit. At this point my hands had started to turn blue. They were like a magic trick. If I was stressed or cold they would turn colors, Red, blue, white. And they would hurt. But the ER doctors just chalked everything up to stress. So home I went, still not knowing what the heck was going on and feeling embarrassed. In hindsight, it was almost a stroke-like, or a seizure-like episode.

As my hands got worse I was diagnosed with Raynaud's disease. My legs became weaker. My joints were hurting like heck, everywhere. I could barely make it up our stairs at the end of the day. At work, I did not think I could finish out a day because of the weakness and fatigue. My fingers hurt, my wrists hurt, and my knees, ankles, and feet hurt. I could not stand on my feet they hurt so badly. When I stood up from a chair I was so stooped over I looked like I was 90 although I was only 54. I walked like Herman Munster. I felt like I was dragging a 500-pound-weight along with me. My primary care provider blamed it all on stress and because it was true that I was under a lot of stress I believed it.

By now I had started having trouble swallowing. I was choking on food, coughing, and could not swallow pills. They dilated my esophagus twice during this period to help me swallow. I had a colonoscopy done for the uncontrollable diarrhea and it showed microscopic colitis called lymphocytic which is also an autoimmune disorder. So I decided I really needed to see a rheumatologist.

After an hour of looking at blood work and labs and examining me the rheumatologist diagnosed me with Scleroderma.

My weakness was getting worse and my fatigue was out of control. The rheumatologist prescribed hydroxychloroquine and also pentoxifylline. That helped with many symptoms but my legs were still getting weaker and my brain felt like mush. I could not speak correctly, couldn't get the words out of my mouth. I would say window for mirror. I started to act differently - not like myself. My short term memory was gone. Sometimes someone would be talking to me and I would not comprehend the words. I would only hear blah, blah, blah.

Then I started having balance issues. I was scared, and felt like I had dementia. I would be in public and if I had to walk down a few stairs I looked like a drunk. I had to hang onto the railing and yet I still tipped and felt like I would fall. I could not make it through a doorway without hitting the wall or door frame.

There was a long period of time where I experienced no feelings. I could not cry, or feel badly about things. It was weird. I was unnerved by this. I was so apathetic. I would know I should be upset or cry, but could not. I also became an angry person and that is not my personality. I felt myself getting angry at work, saying things I would never have said before.

Around this time, my rheumatologist changed my diagnoses to Undifferentiated Connective Tissue Disease (UCTD) with features of scleroderma. He said the medicine he put me on was treating it so quickly he was changing the diagnosis to this. (Now I was really confused.) I felt worse than ever and still I felt no one was listening to me. They just changed my diagnosis once again.

As I went to my primary care provider for help I complained that I had such weird symptoms, the pins and needles in my feet, my legs hurting so bad, not able to do stairs, aching, memory loss, my inability to speak correctly. She responded that she thought it was depression, but also gave me a choice: did I want to see a neurologist, or did I want to start on an antidepressant medication. I told her I wanted to do both, so that is what I did.

I now had an appointment with a neurologist but in between this time my balance got worse, I had mood issues, problems with speech, thought patterns, concentration, and anxiety. I would see things out of my peripheral vision that were not there. I was so tired and I hurt everywhere. I was walking into walls. I would tip standing still. I looked like I was drunk, tipping over, not being able to walk a straight line. I would tip in the shower. I fell a few times for no reason. I dragged my right foot.

So the neurologist started tests: EEG, EMG, MRI, MRA, Nerve Conduction Test, Spinal Taps, Nerve Biopsy and Muscle Biopsy. She diagnosed me with progressive inflammatory myopathy (which is a progressive muscle disease) and peripheral neuropathy with the symptoms of UCTD affecting my central nervous system. My EEG showed nonspecific slowing over the left temporal region, with some focal cortical slowing or dysfunction in that region of an uncertain nature.

At this point I began having episodes that are hard to explain. I would say it would be epileptic in nature in the way they acted. Again I landed back in the hospital, this time for three days, as they ran heart tests because of my weird symptoms. I was driving one day and looked at a stop light and my whole upper body felt like an out-of-body type experience for a lack of a better way of putting it, or like my body was not my own. I was shaking, my brain went to mush, and I felt my arms were too heavy to hold on to the wheel. I waited a few minutes and in very poor judgment decided to try to drive home. When I did get home my husband took me to the ER.

After three days of tests in the hospital they released me, saying my potassium was down at dangerous levels and they felt it was stress and anxiety again. Now I was even more embarrassed. How could this Type A personality, who was never sick, be having all of these weird symptoms yet there was supposedly nothing wrong?

At this time I was on around 30 pills a day for the other disorders. I was put on Imuran for the scleroderma, and carbamazepine for the peripheral neuropathy to name a few. My neurologist knew I was getting worse and she decided to refer me to Mayo for a second opinion, which unfortunately my insurance would not cover. So we went to Northwestern University teaching hospital in Chicago, Illinois. They had Scleroderma specialists and she wanted a second opinion from one of their neurologists regarding the treatments I was getting.

While I was there they did a Thyroid Peroxidase antibody blood test and it came back very high at 1203, with normal being 35 u/ml. When I went back to my neurologist I showed her the results and she did her own blood work. Sure enough, there it was. All the pieces of the HE puzzle came together. I was diagnosed with Hashimoto's Encephalopathy. During this period my cpk was high, as was my creatinine. I was diagnosed with myositis, which is another very rare autoimmune disease.

At my next appointment my neurologist told me it took so long to diagnose the HE because it is very hard to diagnose, being a diagnosis of exclusion. They started me on 1000 mg a day of methylprednisone via IV, as an outpatient, and I did feel better rather quickly. Not perfect, but better. The prednisone caused my blood pressure to go sky high, dangerously so. It caused my cholesterol level to go up and I'm now on meds for that, and they changed my blood pressure meds to regulate the raised blood pressure. But as far as the treatment itself, that was not painful and it was easy.

The tapering dose was a different story. I felt so awful coming off of the prednisone. Every problem I had, every ache in my body was intensified by a factor of ten. This did not last much longer than a week, but it was a heck of a long week. They then raised my Imuran from 150 mg to 200 mg a day to take care of another autoimmune disorder. I did not want to go on daily prednisone because of all the side effects. That is just my wish right now.

When I was first told I had HE I had no clue at all what this was. I looked up every bit of information I could on the internet, and there wasn't much. What I did find led me to believe that I would be treated with prednisone and would be all better. I would go into remission and all my problems would be over. I would be able to walk for distances again, my fatigue would be gone, my brain fog would be better. I would be able to hold an intelligent conversation again. My short term memory would come back. I would not tip anymore. But this was not true for me. I think it is a false hope to tell us HE patients, since it doesn't work out that way for so many of us.

Yes, I am better. I am not reversing my words constantly, although I do still do it. My balance is much better but not perfect. I do not drag my right foot anymore, only if I overdo it or I am stressed. But my fatigue is still bad, my short term memory is still bad, my concentration is still bad. I have no endurance. I just try to accept things as they are.

I have always been the one whose cup is half full and I still am, but there are moments when I remember who I used to be and that makes me sad. But I do appreciate the person I am now. I take time to enjoy little things I never had time for. I make time to stay in contact with my friends and family. I was always so busy working and trying to make a living, but now God has given me no choice in the matter. He has slowed me down.

My neurologist told me back in May of 2011 I needed to quit my job. So I did quit in July of 2011 and it has helped. I know I could not have done it anymore anyway. But having the doctor tell me to do it gave me no option, so that made it a little easier. I have started doing crafts that I had not had time for since I was a young woman. I read, and I talk to my Facebook friends in my health groups, who I find are great support systems for me.

I had a hard time telling my family everything. I have always been the strong one, the one everyone went to, and I did not want to lose that. I did not want anyone to feel sorry for me, or baby me. So I held a lot in for a long time, which was not fair to them. They deserved to know. My doctor kept asking me if I had talked to my family, and whether I was getting support from them. Eventually I did start to give them information. I would send them articles and information on my diagnoses, including the HE. My oldest son had also been encouraging me to set up a blog for all to follow, so with his help I did do that too.

Nine months after the diagnosis of HE I have found peace within myself. I have come to understand myself and my diseases better. I do not panic when I have a day where I tip just standing still, or when I am so exhausted I have to sit in my chair and do handy work. I am learning my pace in life. If I want to do something one day I rest the day before and the day after. It is just the way it is for me. I may vacuum the house and then sit for half an hour to rest, then get up and do dishes, then rest, etc. This is ok with me now. I may nap in the afternoon, or just sit for a few hours to rest. I did feel guilty over this since my husband works very hard, but I have learned to control that guilt. Some days I cannot make supper because of the fatigue but we make do. I also started to go see a physiologist to help handle some of the issues that come along with chronic diseases and pain which I feel has helped. Just recently I started with a pain specialist who I am hoping will help with my constant chronic pain.

I still suffer with problems of forgetting, leaving things on, starting to drive and forgetting where I am going. I have trouble with my eyes with lights. Driving with the street lights sometimes bothers me, making me feel like I may have another out of body feeling. I have strange sensations of itching all over (which could be from the UCTD), but that is the problem: I have no way of knowing which symptom goes with which disorder. I get sharp electrical-type shock pains in my skull that last only a brief second. I have also had this in my leg with the sharp shock light pain from my ankle to my thigh. My legs are weak but this could also be the Myositis, although I know others who have HE who suffer with the same. I have jerking movements in my legs and arms, twitching in my face and eyes. I have incontinence and incomplete emptying. I have strange pains that will affect my toe one day, then my side for three days, then it will hurt my arm, or my groin. My neurologist suggests this is the neuropathy. Last year I had an episode where my jaw froze shut. I could not open it for an entire day, and could only sip things through a straw slid in between my lips. I also have TMJ, and suffer from very dry mouth, skin, eyes and private area. So I never know what is going to happen or when or where.

Hashimoto Encephalitis can cause some very peculiar symptoms, and it's interesting to see that members of our HE group have so many oddities in common, such as reading magazines from the back to the front, writing words that are missing letters, writing sentences that are missing words, getting in the car and not having any idea where we were going to go, leaving things on the stove and forgetting we were cooking. But I know I can live with this because I am living, thanks to my doctors.

I have to thank my great doctors, especially my neurologist Dr. Santillan, as I feel without her aggressive treatment and diagnostic approach I would be in great danger. Autoimmune diseases and disorders are very hard to diagnose and I am so appreciative of my doctors working for me as a team to see me through all of this.

Do I feel I am in remission? It is so hard to say. My numbers are still high, not in the thousands anymore, better but not normal. But it is hard for me to know since I do have so many other issues going on. I feel I am better, but remission, no. I think mine is a very slow progressive process - this is just my own thoughts.

I do feel in my heart that autoimmune diseases do have a tendency to attack people who are under extreme stress, causing our immune system to attack our own bodies. I also believe it tends to run in families, as my mother had thyroid problems, her mother, her sisters. So I hope it stops with me. I also will not be surprised to find out someday that HE runs in families as I look back and see a lot of symptoms I have that mirror symptoms that my deceased mother also suffered with.

Right now, I have vision issues, I am restricted to local driving, and even then sometimes I am hesitant to leave the house and drive. Lights bother me. I have gotten glasses with high transitional lenses to help with the changes in light. It is like my brain cannot handle the switches from regular light to bright light. I have days I feel very confused, I am always tired, some days much worse than others. My brain will get overloaded very easily and makes me feel foggy or like it may explode. I always have pressure in my head or a numbness feeling. Some days I cannot figure out what to do with the simplest of things, for instance looking at two pieces of paper in hand and not knowing what to do first. I have to think for a few seconds to say the right word, really concentrate on it before I speak. But all and all, I just am so happy to be alive.

Medications I am on at present are:

- Amlodopine 10 mg tablet for blood pressure and Raynauds; it is a calcium channel blocker
- Aspirin 81 mg tablet one a day
- Fluticasone Nasal spray
- Furosemide 40 mg tablet one a day for water pill
- Levothyroxine 100 mcg pill one a day for hypothyroidism
- Estrace cream for vaginal dryness
- Levocetirizine 5 mg tablet one a day for allergies
- Azathioprine 50 mg (just changed to 3) was 4 (Imuran)
- Lorazapam .05 mg 1-2 tablets three times a day for anxiety
- Lexapro 20 mg once a day for depression
- Carbamazepine 100 mg 2 tablets twice a day for neuropathy
- Hydrocodone APAP 5-325 mg tablets 3 times a day for pain
- Omeprazole 20 mg capsules twice a day for reflux

- D 1.25MG 50,000 units one every other week
- Klor-con M20 Tablet 1 tab every day (potassium)
- Lisinopril 5 mg tablet for high blood pressure (My pressure started to rise in Aug 2012 and was fluctuating so this was added to bring it down. This is an Ace Inhibitor.

I have also been on Nuvigil for concentration, Pentoxifylline for Raynauds, and Hydroxychloroquine for the Scleroderma. Also for the autoimmune colitis I have been on Aasacol EC 400 mg 6 a day along with Pepto Bismal tablets 6 a day which right now I do not need any of these.

My diagnoses are:

- Raynaud's
- Hypothyroid
- UCTD with features of scleroderma
- High blood pressure
- Lymphocytic colitis
- Myositis
- Peripheral neuropathy
- Esophagus reflux
- Photosensitive
- Hearing issues
- Myopathy underlined by autoimmune diseases
- Neuromuscular involvement
- Bladder issues

That's my HE story. But for me, it wasn't enough to just get a diagnosis and find treatment. This affliction was, I believe, an opportunity for me to do something more than just help myself get better.

Like Anji, when I received my HE diagnosis my initial reaction was: I have what? Rare? Can you spell that please? Can you repeat that slower?

I went on the internet looking, seeking, hungry for information. I found maybe two articles that were very out-of-date and all the information said pretty much the same thing: I would have no problem after I received IV infusions of meythlprednisone. I would be back to normal, would be able to work and so on. Well, to my surprise this was not true. I went back to the internet again to search some more. This time I crossed my fingers and went to Facebook, where I found the site started by Anji, which is a wonderful site for those of us diagnosed with HE. And I found out I was not alone - there were others like me, still having many problems.

This made me think, how many others that are diagnosed cannot find up to date information? Patients who are searching for others to compare themselves with, wishing for a place to share stories and experiences? Hashimoto's Encephalopathy can present so differently in different patients, but there are so many things in common that we do share, and that I think we should be aware of.

So talking to a fellow HE suffer (Nicola) one day, I brought up the idea of writing a book of patient stories so that others who may be diagnosed will not have to be as confused as I was. Nicola thought it was a great idea also, and at that point we started making plans for our book on HE.

That is how the book idea began. We soon started to ask if members of the Facebook group would like to share their stories to help others that are diagnosed with HE, and thankfully we received a lot of positive feedback on the idea.

Nicola and I cannot take credit for this book. The people who took the time to write out their stories are the ones to thank. Without them you would not have this book in your hands.

I hope this book can help others see what we have gone through, and help them to know what to realistically expect from a diagnosis of HE. I know my case is a little more involved than others, which made it even harder to diagnose, because of the other autoimmune diseases. But in telling my story I felt it was important for me to start at the beginning of my process with autoimmune diseases so other patients and physicians could see what could happen, and did happen, and how not to let other diagnoses cloud the vision of a diagnosis of HE. My neurologist did say to me that when God was handing down autoimmune diseases he decided to give them all to you.

I hope this book will help others the way we intended it to. I hope it calms fears, help patients become more educated, makes it easier to find up-to-date medical articles on HE, and helps the loved ones of HE patients find answers.

Nicola

My HE story begins in December 2010, when I started to notice I was having difficulty with concentration, memory, and word finding. I was a successful environmental attorney at a major, national law firm, and the largest part of my practice involved researching and analyzing state and federal environmental regulations and the court cases interpreting them, and then applying my analysis to my clients' cases. Needless to say, concentration, memory and word finding were extremely important, and when I began to notice problems with these things I was a little worried. But I put it off to over-work and started keeping my office door closed during working hours. I posted a sign on the door encouraging colleagues and staff to feel free to enter, explaining that the door was merely closed to minimize distraction.

On the morning of February 11, 2011, I was sitting at my desk, immersed in writing an appellate brief, when I suddenly experienced severe confusion. At the same time, the vision disappeared from my right eye. I was used to having migraines that sometimes presented with a visual disturbance, but this was nothing like a migraine.

I decided to go talk to my secretary but had trouble walking the hundred or so feet to her desk. My balance was off, and I felt terribly weak. When I got to her desk I was unable to speak. I was aware of some vague right-sided weakness, and I was feeling more confused by the moment. She asked me what was wrong, and when I couldn't answer she quickly took action.

I couldn't remember my husband's phone number, or my doctor's name. Everything was going completely blank inside my head. I didn't lose consciousness, but suddenly found myself at the hospital, not entirely sure how I'd gotten there.

There I was evaluated for a possible stroke, but tests showed no evidence of one, and the next day I was released with a diagnosis of complicated migraine, or, less possibly, a TIA. I felt a little better when I got home, and although I could speak my speech was slow and labored. Everything around me seemed to be happening in slow motion. I felt like I was – metaphorically speaking – slogging through thick, deep mud, both cognitively and physically.

I tried to return to work a few days later but when I sat down at my desk I could not figure out what to do with the materials in front of me. I attempted to read the appellate brief I had been writing a few days earlier but couldn't make out what it said. I could pick out words but wasn't sure of their meaning, and I couldn't follow a sentence from beginning to end.

My family physician ordered a couple of weeks off work to see if things would get back to normal for me, and I followed up with the neurologist who had seen me while I was in the hospital. Unfortunately, things didn't go back to normal, and an abnormal EEG about a month later led the neurologist to prescribe Tegretol, which he later switched to Keppra in April. My symptoms continued to worsen.

I was having periodic seizure-like episodes involving intense confusion, the complete loss of ability to speak, and muscle rigidity, sometimes including facial paralysis. I was also having a terrible problem with my memory, concentration, and language ability. My speech was halting and effortful, and I regularly used the wrong words for things. I experienced debilitating fatigue, headaches, periodic tremors, muscle twitching and jerking, and joint pain. My balance was terrible, and I kept walking into things, and worse still, falling.

A particularly upsetting symptom was a problem I began having with my throat. It would suddenly constrict, randomly, and I would simultaneously experience something like the effect of "ear popping" one sometimes feels when encountering a change in altitude. If I happened to be speaking at the time, the pitch of my voice would suddenly rise until the constriction stopped. It was terribly embarrassing, and at the same time terrifying.

In April 2011 my neurologist ordered a 48-hour video EEG (which turned into a 72-hour EEG) to be administered in our hometown hospital. The video EEG showed "occasional rhythmic discharges" and background slowing, but no evidence of epileptic seizures. Nonetheless, I was now having seizure-like events multiple times a day in the hospital. I began hallucinating, believing there was an old woman in a rocking chair in the corner of my hospital room, knitting away. I heard phantom sounds: strange music, ringing telephones, and peculiar electronic noises. Worst of all, I began having horrifying olfactory hallucinations. I was engulfed with the stench of an odor like that of a rotting animal corpse (something I'd encountered a couple of times in my life when I was young). No matter what I did, I couldn't escape the smell. The only thing that helped – and my family still finds this hilarious – was if I buried my face in my husband's armpit. Perhaps it was the reptilian brain at work, but that was the only escape for me…inhaling that very personal, human odor.

The neurologist who was "treating me" (and I use that term loosely, given that he did so little) decided that what I really needed was a psychiatrist, and he told my husband he was releasing me from the hospital with a psychiatric referral. At this point, my daughter – who works in health care – came to the rescue and demanded that the hospital get another neurologist in to see me right away.

They obliged, and after a brief interview that neurologist ordered thyroid antibody testing, and low and behold, we were on our way to a diagnosis. He had me transferred via ambulance that night from our hometown hospital to the University of Illinois Medical Center in Chicago. There, doctors finally performed a full neurological examination – something my neurologist at home had never done. They found I had hyperreflexia, and a positive Romberg response. When I attempted to draw a clock, I began by putting the number 1 at the top, where the 12 should go, and was perplexed when I ran out of places for numbers when I got to 11. (I squeezed in a tiny little 12 between the 11 and the 1, figuring it must surely go in there somewhere!)

Doctors at the U of I ran countless tests, including an MRI, CT scan, a lumbar puncture, and of course loads of blood tests. My thyroid antibodies were re-tested. In addition to multiple neurological examinations, I was also examined by an endocrinologist, who confirmed that I had Hashimoto's Thyroiditis. The doctors attempted to do a PET scan but were unable to get the necessary authorization, so instead they ordered a SPECT scan, which showed, among other things, hypoperfusion throughout my left cerebral hemisphere.

The U of I hospital was a mixed blessing. On one hand I finally got thorough testing and ultimately my diagnosis of Steroid Responsive Encephalopathy Associated with Thyroiditis. But at the same time, my team of doctors there had a mixed response to me. While some were convinced I had HE/SREAT, others preferred a psychiatric diagnosis – despite my abnormal test results.

One of them told me I had "hypergraphia," because by this time I was obsessively writing notes all day. What they didn't understand was that because my memory was virtually nonexistent, without my notes I never had any idea what had happened on a given day. (They told me Tolstoy was hypergraphic too, and suggested it could mean Temporal Lobe Epilepsy, which wouldn't necessarily show up on an EEG.) They couldn't fathom my desperation to hang on to my experiences of the day, so my endless scribbling looked like a strange, compulsive disorder.

Despite my severe memory and concentration problems, doctors seemed to want to focus primarily on my speech problems, perhaps because that was something they could observe, unlike my severe memory and concentration impairment, both of which were invisible of course. In the same way, they liked checking my balance and gait because this, too, could be objectively quantified.

In any case, I got the treatment I needed. After five-and-a-half days of high dose IV steroids (1000 mg per day), my speech returned to near-normal and they were elated. I also rapidly regained the ability to recite back to them extremely long strings of numbers or words - forwards or backwards. I could read and understand written material, and the hallucinations stopped.

Despite the initial relief I got from symptoms with the IV steroid treatment, my symptoms returned during the subsequent steroid-tapering process. Over the next year and a half I saw a series of physicians, none of whom were able to help me regain my former level of function, although they never tried giving me another round of IV steroids which, in retrospect, might have been extremely helpful.

Reluctantly, I “retired” from my law firm, despite the fact that I was only 55. There was simply no way I could function as an attorney with recurring episodes of transient global amnesia and mental confusion, impaired speech, very limited reading ability, and periodic seizure-like or stroke-like events during which I became disoriented and unable to communicate.

For me, having HE has been like being trapped in a Kafka story. My life was – in an instant - turned upside down, my career stripped away. My ability to reflect and to engage in contemplation suddenly vanished, taking with it my sense of personal identity. Where my inner life had once been rich with vibrant intellectual curiosity, there was now only deafening silence inside my head. I couldn't articulate my thoughts – when I had any – with any clarity, and I regularly found myself spouting only nonsensical gibberish when I tried to speak. I had lost virtually all my stamina, careening between exhaustion and insomnia, and was so overwhelmed by the visual and auditory input from a visit to the local grocery store that I stopped trying to go along with my husband on shopping trips.

I would boot up my computer and find myself unable to remember how to open an email, how to reply to a message, or sometimes, how to shut the darned thing down. I forgot for weeks at a time that Facebook had a "news feed" function, despite the fact that this is how I had regularly communicated with friends.

One thing I found perplexing was the response of most physicians to these symptoms throughout the first few months of my suffering. They would assure me that I was actually fine, there was nothing wrong with my brain, and announced my neuropsych exam showed I was functioning at an "average" level (or, at least "low-average" in terms of cognition). The advice they gave, all too often, was to relax, accept that it might be part of the aging process, and "see a psychiatrist." Kafkaesque indeed, for someone who had been a highly skilled attorney just months earlier.

The one physician who never wavered in his support was my primary care physician, Dr. Ralph Everson, to whom I remain eternally grateful. He had known me before I got sick and could see the drastic change, whereas those physicians who met me after I was impaired had no real frame of reference. He has always been supportive and helpful, and I feel certain there is a special place in heaven for physicians like him.

Ultimately, I was fortunate enough to find Dr. Franczak, a memory specialist at Froedtert Hospital in Milwaukee. She listened to me. She heard what I was saying, and truly understood the devastation I faced. She validated my concern about the serious hazards associated with most of the available treatments for HE, and let me know that she would leave it up to me to inform her when my symptoms were bad enough to require pharmaceutical intervention. Finally I have a neurologist who seems to really "get" what I am saying. She supports my decision to live with vastly diminished cognition and memory, and impaired speech, in order to avoid the terrible side effects of ongoing immunosuppression, at least for now.

These days I am cultivating first and foremost the art of PATIENCE. That is clearly one of the important life-lessons for me in all this. Patience has been my nemesis since I was a child, and I've been given experience after experience and challenge after challenge in my life that seem to have been designed to help me acquire that elusive trait. I'm better at it now than I was ten years ago, twenty years ago, thirty years ago, but I still have a long, long way to go in learning to be patient, especially with myself.

Like others, my illness has made me aware of just how much it means to have loving family and friends. I am so grateful for my incredible husband Steven (36 years of marriage and a love that's deeper than ever), our three grown children (Jesse, Sarah, and Danny), our dear, departed daughter Laura (see you in Paradise!), my darling new granddaughter, Harper, and our three dogs, not to mention the greatest friends in the world. Without them, I'm not sure how I would have kept going when things were at their darkest.

But the greatest gift in all this – my silver lining – is the chance to take my devastating experience with HE and use it for good in the world. I have been given the precious opportunity to use what remains of my research and writing ability to search for new information about HE, to create a log of scientific articles so that others who are researching the disease can more easily locate the latest information.

I had the great good fortune to come across the Facebook community started by Anji Hogan-Fesler early on in my HE journey. There I found a place to commiserate with others, to share treatment options and names of physicians, to cry over the sorrows of HE, and to laugh over the quirky and ever-surprising antics of "Hashi-Brain."

At about the same time I stumbled across an amazing WordPress webpage – "henotebook" – that had been put together by another HE patient – a woman named Allison - a former electrical engineer who dubbed herself "Scientist Seeking." (Her story appears later in this book.) Allison and I collaborated to update her page, and soon I was adding new citations for scientific articles about HE to the page almost monthly, as research continued to pour in from scientists around the world (on days when my brain was cooperating and I could remember how to work the computer).

When Susan Foley, who I'd met online, suggested that we collect as many stories of HE patients as we could and put them into a book, the idea clicked with me right away. And Anji, beautiful soul that she is, nurtured our effort and encouraged members of the Facebook community to share their experiences with us.

My former law firm, Hinshaw & Culbertson, generously provided the legal assistance needed to form a nonprofit: the Hashimoto's Encephalopathy SREAT Alliance ("HESA"). I launched the HESA website with the help of a family friend, Toby Cryns, and began reaching out to other encephalopathy-related organizations around the world. Meanwhile, Susan and

I kept plugging along, collecting stories and working through the myriad details of book publishing until finally, after two years of hard work, it was done.

What follows next are the stories of HE patients contributed by members of the Facebook HE community, the E-Global community at Inspire.com, and the HELPS group at Topica.com.

The first of these stories, by "Shari," is the longest. In it, Shari not only narrates her personal journey, she also offers detailed advice for patients, family members, and treaters based on what she has learned.

Shari (age at diagnosis: 41)

I still don't know exactly where my more garden-variety health problems ended and Hashimoto's Encephalopathy officially began, but after over two dozen doctors and one heck of a goose chase, here's what we think we know:

Prior to my HE diagnosis, I'd had chronic allergies and migraines, frequent infections, anemia, endometriosis, and a variety of other 'ordinary' troubles accompanied by major fatigue despite a lot of sleep. I followed the doctor's instructions to manage each of these, but still knew 'something wasn't right'. I didn't realize until I got a copy of all my medical records that I'd had Hashimoto's thyroid disease for years but it had been overlooked.

In the meantime, I took lots of vitamins and used a sinus rinse to help keep infections at bay. I lived on Advil, Excedrin, Benadryl and Sudafed, popped a lot of antibiotics (and probiotics!), and slept a lot. I still felt awful most of the time. I ended up with erosions in my intestines from all the pain medicine, and the Sudafed may have contributed to several bouts of ischemic colitis. One by one, I lost the ability to keep up with various things in my life – from friendships, to opening the mail, to taking care of my personal appearance. I was able to stay afloat at my job through late starts and a lot of unplanned work from home, but my employer's patience was wearing thin.

After a particular string of infections in late 2011, I found myself having a lot of weird cognitive problems. For long stretches of time, I'd be unable to figure out how to do the job for which I'd been winning awards for 16 years – I'd sit down at my computer and nothing at all would happen, like my brain was a computer that wouldn't boot up. Despite years of 'safe driver' awards, I crashed into a parked car right in front of my house. When I asked my primary doctor what might be wrong, she read me a questionnaire on depression. I tried another doctor, and he said that I didn't need any tests – I just needed to stop taking all those stupid vitamins and exercise 30 minutes a day and I'd be fine. A chiropractor who was also a naturopath picked up indications of immune and autoimmune dysfunction, but couldn't pinpoint the cause. I got a copy of my old medical records and learned my TSH had been signaling trouble since at least 1999.

I got on thyroid replacement hormone in February of 2012, and my brain gradually came back online over the next couple of months. I don't know if that episode of cognitive problems was due to hypothyroidism, or if it was my first recognizable bout of HE. (A literature review published in 2006 indicated that 17% of cases of HE resolve with levothyroxine alone, acknowledging that those cases might have been destined to resolve spontaneously, which can also happen.)

With my mind working again, I thought we'd finally cracked the code, but the success was short lived. Perhaps triggered by my first bout of ischemic colitis in May of 2012, things started sliding again – and getting weirder. My interpersonal interactions became progressively more confusing. I often couldn't follow what people were saying, and couldn't parse implied instructions. I didn't pick up on normal social cues, and I got yelled at for failing to 'read the room' or 'read between the lines' in situations where there were serious business consequences. People got mad at me – a lot. I got my first-ever inadequate performance review at work from an angry boss who thought I could only be underperforming on purpose. He kept insisting "I know you're smarter than that!" He yelled that if he received one more complaint about me, 'corrective action would be taken, do I make myself clear!'

I tried harder. Everything I did took too long – if I could do it at all. I didn't understand what was going wrong, and didn't even know what questions to ask. I was baffled, humiliated and terrified that I couldn't figure out how to do things I had known how to do for years. My husband was extremely frustrated with me and with the situation.

I was desperate for ANYTHING that might help me 'pull myself together'. We checked our home for mold and radon. Despite finding no issues and having a fancy whole-house filter on the furnace, we set up three medical grade air purifiers and a digital radon detector. We got a pair of exercise bikes and I tried to get some 'proper exercise' though I could barely turn the pedals – since I couldn't rule that out until I'd tried it. We got a special blue light that's supposed to help regulate circadian rhythms, and set it to turn on just before the alarm went off in the morning. I took over a dozen prescription vitamins. I started doing Reiki (a form of energy healing) on myself daily. I researched possibilities online and tried to find a new doctor who might be able to help.

In August I asked an immunologist for assistance troubleshooting my errant immune system. The test results showed some immunoglobulin subfactors were a bit low, so she prescribed an 'immune challenge' – I was to get the pneumonia vaccine and see if my body could make antibodies. Things unraveled quickly after that. I'll never know if it was a reaction to the vaccine, some weird virus that kicked me when I was down, or the blossoming of something that was already underway.

The Really Weird Days

At first I thought it was just another weird illness – fever, headache, body aches, severe fatigue, abdominal pain, diarrhea, and loss of appetite. I was afraid of losing my job because of the health and performance issues I'd been having, so I pushed myself to go to work anyhow. I had recently been moved under a new boss, and she sent me home because I was twitching and shaking uncontrollably. She thought I must have the chills.

I got a same-day appointment with a kind and thorough doctor who had never seen me before. He did a complete blood count and tested for influenza, metabolic problems, electrolyte imbalance, and possible worsening hypothyroid, but nothing jumped out to explain the symptoms. My TSH was normal at 2.2. I'd gotten numerous mosquito bites at an outdoor wedding a couple of weeks prior, so he drew blood to test for West Nile virus. Unfortunately, it turned out there was a shortage of West Nile tests available, so the test went on back order and I went home.

Over the weekend, the jerking of my muscles (which I later learned was called myoclonus) got a lot worse. My limbs flailed and my trunk muscles pulled me into the fetal position over and over again. It was like every part of me had its own personal case of the hiccups. It was constant whenever I was awake, but cold, stress, or being startled really sent it into high gear. I told my husband it was alright, because the muscle jerks didn't hurt. I didn't get up much, but when I did I used a blue ski pole to steady myself when the myoclonus knocked me off my feet, or when my legs just went out from under me. We called it my Weeble stick (so I could wobble but not fall down). I slept over 20 hours a day. I started slurring my words. For all that was happening, this typical chronic worrier with a very busy brain really didn't have many thoughts or feelings about any of it.

The myoclonus wasn't as intense Monday morning and my fever was down. The "I'm afraid of losing my job" devil kept tugging at my sleeve, so I decided to test my ability to function by driving my husband the six blocks to the train station on his way to work. (I have since learned that uncharacteristically poor judgment can be one of the many symptoms of HE.) When I started the car, the air conditioning blasted me with cold air and triggered a major bout of myoclonus. I panicked and started hitting everything in the car. I couldn't figure out how the controls worked. My husband was alarmed but I was not listening. I used all of my will to figure out how to reverse the car. There was a garbage truck working the opposite side of the street, and I could not figure out how to get around it. I pulled into oncoming traffic and froze. My husband kept telling me to reverse but I couldn't do it. I just sat there, right in front of my own house, until the other cars reversed out of my path. I finally 'got it' that something was really wrong.

I sent my husband off to walk to the train and called my parents crying. This was one of three times during this illness that I cried (which is a bit odd for someone who's been known to be moved to tears watching a children's vitamin commercial). The same-day doctor I had seen the previous week instructed us to go to the emergency room to expedite getting the right tests run. When we got there, I couldn't read the clock face. I knew it should mean something to me, but I couldn't figure out how to use the symbols to tell me what time it was. All my muscles jerked, my head hurt, and my abdomen hurt. I was having a lot of trouble putting my thoughts into words or finding the words I wanted. I kept trying to explain that my mind was slow and fuzzy and things were confusing. My family could readily tell I wasn't myself, but my basic neurological exam was within normal limits and I didn't sound alarmingly 'abnormal' or impaired to strangers. To be on the safe side, they admitted me so more tests could be run, including an expedited West Nile. I was placed in an isolation room in case it was something contagious.

Each of the next four days a variety of different doctors did the rounds. I tried to explain how my mind wasn't working right, but I couldn't really get anyone to understand. Mostly I slept. When my family called, I told them I didn't want any company. I didn't have any news or thoughts or feelings, and I just wanted to sleep. The hospital had Wi-Fi and a few times I tried to look up West Nile or other terms that had been batted around, but I couldn't really wrap my head around the sea of words that appeared. I'd get a few words in and trail off. Later I'd realize that I'd just been staring at nothing for a long time. I was so tired. At school I'd always tested seven years or more above grade level in reading, but suddenly I couldn't read more than a sentence or two. I thought maybe I was just wiped out from whatever bug I had.

Each day I saw different neurologists, nurses, and hospitalists. I kept passing the tests the doctors gave me – did I know my name and where I was, could I name basic items in a line drawing. They performed other standard neurological tests like asking me to follow their finger with my eyes. They ordered brain and spinal MRIs, an EEG, a lumbar puncture, and blood work. My lab test results were largely normal. Much later, I later learned the EEG was 'obscured' by the myoclonus but didn't suggest epilepsy. The spinal MRIs were essentially normal. The brain MRI showed 'small areas of increased signal intensity within the left frontal and parietal lobe white matter and pons, nonspecific', but it wasn't clear when the damage had appeared. It hadn't been present in an MRI done during a severe migraine episode I'd had ten years earlier, but the damage didn't light up further when they injected contrast dye, which the report said meant the damage might not be brand new. But I learned all of that later; in the hospital I was simply reassured that my MRI was 'normal for my age', which at the time was 40.

While I was in the hospital, I didn't know what all they were testing for, and I kept asking if anyone could give me a copy of any of the results. Each person I asked said they were nothing to worry about. Someone told me that my expedited West Nile test results came back normal. One of the nurses finally gave me a one-page grid with some of my blood test results. I will be eternally grateful to her, as that printout ultimately turned out to be the key to getting diagnosis and treatment. The next nurse I asked for information told me that it was the hospital's policy that only the medical records department or the too-busy doctor who ordered the individual test was allowed to provide me copies of any records. The nurse who informed me of the rule brought me the official form to request copies of my results from the medical records department. It took over two months for the records I requested that day to show up at my house.

In the meantime, the neurologist-of-the-day discharged me with an anti-seizure medication prescription, an information sheet about myoclonus, and instructions to make an appointment to follow up with a neurologist in a week or so. He offered no theories as to what they thought was causing my troubles, and no mention of the cognitive problems I kept trying to get someone to understand were the 'real issue' to me.

My mom picked me up from the hospital. We called the neurologist's office on the way home, and were told the next available appointment was over a month away. At home, we googled things from the blood test printout to try to understand what they might mean. The results listed on the printout indicated that my spinal fluid showed slightly elevated protein and glucose, and my blood mild anemia. The only thing that was really out of whack was something called 'Anti-microsomal Ab', also known as 'anti-TPO antibodies' against the thyroid. Mine were 2,906. The lab's normal range was less than 60. We googled anti-TPO and myoclonus, and up popped a Wikipedia article on Hashimoto's Encephalopathy.

I left a message at the neurologist's office asking if the antibodies, cognitive problems and myoclonus suggested that Hashimoto's Encephalopathy might be a possibility. I got an after-hours call to be at the office at 8 AM the next day. My dad agreed to drive me to the appointment. As we set out for the doctor's office, he handed me the map he had printed off the internet and asked me which direction to go. I stared at the paper, but even though I was in a town I'd lived in for over 30 years I couldn't figure out how to use the picture to tell us where to go. Dad took over navigating and got us there.

By sheer luck, it turned out that the neurologist who had ordered the antibody test at the hospital was the one with whom I'd gotten the appointment. He issued a tentative diagnosis of Hashimoto's Encephalopathy, and agreed it was not necessary for me to take the anti-seizure medication. He promised my dad he would 'quarterback' my treatment, which would probably include steroids. The immunologist I'd seen in August confirmed that she'd defer to whatever treatment the neurologist recommended. The neurologist said he just wanted me to see an endocrinologist colleague to confirm that this was the right approach before starting steroid treatment. I was given an endo appointment for 8 AM the following day.

My dad brought me to the next doctor's appointment too. When I first met with the endocrinologist, he said he didn't believe Hashimoto's Encephalopathy existed. (Later, I learned that many endocrinologists don't believe that thyroid antibodies cross the blood-brain barrier and attack the brain, and that HE patients' symptoms therefore have nothing to do with the thyroid – especially since not everyone with thyroid antibodies gets HE, and since HE symptom intensity generally doesn't correlate to thyroid antibody levels. Rather than saying no illness existed, he was actually suggesting that HE was a misnomer, and that I had 'some other illness' in addition to the thyroid antibodies.) Even though I am usually Miss Mouse with doctors, I got uncharacteristically agitated. I thought he was suggesting I imagined all of my symptoms, but even still, my reaction in his office was out of character. On my visit summary sheet, he coded the diagnosis as "Encephalopathy, unspecified" and wrote that it would be appropriate to treat for possible SREAT (steroid responsive encephalopathy with associated thyroiditis, which is what endocrinologists tend to call Hashimoto's Encephalopathy).

Things were moving so fast. My mom was scared, but I was relieved. I finally had an explanation for the weird things that had been happening, and a plan to fix them. I thought things would be better soon, and I sent a message to my boss.

Shortly afterward, the neurologist called. He said maybe I wasn't actually 'sick enough' to have Hashimoto's Encephalopathy, and he wanted to send me to a 'tertiary research facility' for a second opinion. He then mentioned that it was a movement disorders clinic that he was referring me to. I was perplexed and frustrated, because it sounded to me like he was minimizing the idea of cognitive problems and it also meant delays in getting well and getting back to work. I still followed his instructions, and spent the next two weeks going in circles trying to get the HMO insurance forms successfully faxed from the neurologist's office to the clinic. In the end, my dad called Customer Service at the 'tertiary research facility', and the woman with whom he spoke was somehow able to get the matter resolved. An appointment was finally set.

While all that was going on, I experienced 6 hours of severe double vision one evening, and was advised by the neurologist on call at my regular doctor's office to go to the emergency room. I was admitted, and an MRI was performed in the morning. They told me it was unchanged from the previous MRI and sent me home. This would turn out to be the first of many prolonged episodes of double vision.

Later at the movement disorders clinic, I passed the Mini Mental State Exam and other tests. The doctors at the clinic said my symptoms might be due to HE, but that they didn't have much experience with HE so they weren't sure. They also told me I should really be in a coma or at the very least be unable to walk or talk for it to be HE, unless it was a very 'atypical presentation'. Like all the doctors before them, they didn't rule out HE, they didn't commit to a diagnosis or treatment, and they passed me on to someone else for another opinion. And like all the doctors before them, they were skeptical about whether I was genuinely experiencing any cognitive problems.

As I accumulated my medical records and session notes from the various doctors, I found phrases like 'age-appropriate cognition', 'cannot rule out a psychogenic cause' and 'possible functional overlay'. So it's little wonder the doctors at the movement disorders clinic just wanted to order more tests – evoked potentials to see if the myoclonus was originating in the brain or the spinal cord, a neuropsych evaluation to rule out cognitive deterioration, and another endocrinologist's opinion (even though endocrinologists are rarely the ones to diagnose or treat HE).

Because I had an HMO, each new test required a separate insurance referral from the original neurologist. I figured that was okay, because the neurologist had already promised my dad he would be my quarterback. For reasons unknown, the movement disorders clinic didn't send their results back to the referring neurologist, and he never followed up with them. In hindsight, I think the original neurologist probably believed he had fully handed me off to the clinic, but with an HMO that isn't possible. When I found out he hadn't seen the results, I got the clinic to send him a copy and thought surely the necessary referrals would follow. I got an email from the referring neurologist saying he agreed with their recommendations, but he still never completed the referrals that would have allowed me to follow through on them. Everyone thought someone else was managing my care – which ultimately meant no one was.

In the meantime, things were getting worse, with episodes like me walking outside in my underwear without realizing it, or not being able to figure out how to use the microwave I've had for over a decade. I broke down in tears one day because my pants were falling down and I couldn't get my arms to work to pull them up. During this time, no one thought they were my doctor.

Throughout all of this, Mom kept everyone updated via Facebook so I didn't have to. When I was able to look at the posts, I could see that people were upset and concerned, but it all seemed far away somehow. I'm so grateful for all of the prayers and messages of support and encouragement people sent. Even during the dark times, I did not feel alone.

Friends and family started to network for someone who might be able to help me. They were looking for a neurologist who had experience with HE, and eventually I was connected with the wonderful doctors at University of Chicago. I emailed them with the lab results that made us suspect HE and asked if they would take my case. Fortunately, they did.

As hypothyroidism and certain types of migraines can cause cognitive and neurological problems, the U of C doctors started there, to see what symptoms were left over once those two illnesses were properly managed. The endocrinologist adjusted my thyroid replacement hormone to keep my TSH below 2.5, which ultimately required two and a half times the levothyroxine I'd been on. My infections, bleeding sinuses, severe bodily pain and constipation-so-bad-I-bled disappeared. The neurologist put me on Verapamil, and my daily migraines were gone. We waited a bit to see what impact any of this might have on the cognitive and neurological problems. Unfortunately, they persisted.

During this time the naturopath chiropractor had just come back from a conference, and asked me to do a series of hand movements she described as 'fist knife flat'. I was completely unable to do the sequence correctly, no matter how many times in a row I attempted it. She said it indicated brain dysfunction, but I don't recall exactly what type. I only recently learned that the hand movements are called the 'Luria sequence', and difficulty performing them reveals left frontal lobe dysfunction.

Not long after failing the Luria test, I finally got the results of the formal neuropsych tests recommended by the movement disorders clinic five months previously. They showed frontal lobe impairment, and over 40 IQ points lost. I learned that frontal lobe issues could explain the problems I'd been experiencing with attention and awareness, and that attention problems could be what had led to memories failing to be recorded. Frontal lobe dysfunction could also explain the changes in social awareness and emotional self-regulation, as well as why my mind was so often blank unless an external stimulus poked it. It could explain why my vocabulary was unaffected, but it was still so hard to get my thoughts into the right words. It could explain why I hadn't been able to process and react to my environment properly, and why I got confused so easily – and so much else. I started seeing a cognitive rehabilitation specialist who recognized the signs of frontal lobe impairment immediately, understood without explanation the kinds of troubles these issues could cause in daily living, and was able to recommend compensating and management strategies.

Ten months after I was first hospitalized, a course of prednisone was finally tried – 40 mg a day for two weeks to switch off genes, then 15 mg a day for a few months. I am currently tapering down from that dosage. Within a couple of days of starting the steroids, I felt like 'myself' again. It actually felt like my frozen brain was thawing. I was aware of people and things around me again. I could do the Luria sequence. I had thoughts and feelings. I could crack jokes and laugh. I wanted to write creatively again – and I could. My husband was elated that I was 'back', and upon seeing me again the cognitive rehabilitation specialist commented that I was a completely different person. I got authorization to return to work and by the time all the paperwork was completed, I was back at my job a year to the day after I'd first gone on medical leave.

Looking Back

I don't actually remember a lot from during the illness. Many days the only thing I managed to do during the short amount of time I was awake was watch a little solar-powered plastic flower on the window ledge flap its leaves. I used medical records, correspondence with doctors, and information from family and friends along with my limited memories to piece all of this together. Below, I'll try to describe some of the big things that changed when I got sick, and give enough detail for those who want to compare to their own experiences. I'll try to break things into logical categories based on my best understanding – bearing in mind that I'm not a doctor.

1. Neurological Issues

a. Myoclonus – The myoclonic jerks have varied in intensity and frequency. Over time it happened most with my left arm and leg, but also frequently included my right limbs and abdominal / trunk / neck muscles. Sometimes my muscles would flex, sometimes they would fling my limbs out. During periods when the myoclonus was more intense, I had a very exaggerated startle reflex, and even mild surprise would often trigger or intensify the myoclonus. My husband and one of the hospital doctors confirmed the myoclonic jerks didn't happen while I was sleeping. Early in the illness, the myoclonus would be intense even when I was resting in a chair or lying awake in bed. It generally got worse with stress, cold, 'fighting off a bug', or fatigue. Magnesium supplementation may have helped calm it a little, but it's hard to be sure of cause and effect. Sometimes just prior to muscle contractions I would feel a very brief surge of electrical activity in the area that would jerk, like the feeling just before you shiver if a chill runs down your spine. Sometimes there would be no warning. A couple of times my legs spontaneously gave out from under me while just standing in the kitchen; this may have been 'negative myoclonus'. I have had a couple of minor relapses since starting steroids, and these are really the only times I experience myoclonus now.

b. Other Involuntary Movements – The fingers on both hands – especially the outer few – would curl, extend, and twitch without permission. I'd get buzzing / electric shock / something-crawling-under-the-skin feelings in my face, especially around mouth, usually while in bed, totally calm and at rest. My eyes would feel 'flickery'. These things still happen from time to time.

c. Coordination Problems – I've never had the dexterity of a neurosurgeon, but I had noticeable coordination changes when I'd go through a 'flare'. I'd drop the same thing over and over again, such as a fork, the toothpaste, or a paper I was holding. I'd knock things over more during activities of daily living. My hands glitched a lot when I'd try to type, resulting in wrong characters, out of order characters, missing words, double words, accidentally overwriting things, etc. My hands glitched a lot when I handwrote things too – letters came out in the wrong order, and there were missing letters, extra letters, extra strokes, and missing strokes. All of it was messier. It happened most with cursive or all caps printing, and for some reason it seemed easier to control mixed case printing.

d. Speech Problems – When I could speak, syllables often came out in wrong order and I sometimes stammered, especially if conversation went on for any length of time or I was beginning to fatigue. On 'bad days', I would slur my words pretty badly or get nonsense syllables in place of some of the syllables I was trying to say. Sometimes I could only get the same nonsense syllable over and over and over again and nothing else. I would constantly forget what I was saying in the middle of saying it, especially but not just if there was any distraction.

e. Vertigo – I experienced intense and prolonged bouts of vertigo, especially but not only when lying down.

f. Double Vision – I had numerous episodes of double vision lasting anywhere from a few minutes to six hours. The vision in each eye individually was clear; I just couldn't reconcile things into a single image.

g. Altered Knee Reflexes – Throughout most of the illness, my knee reflexes have been normal when I'm doing well, and 'brisk' when I am doing poorly. The doctor who finally diagnosed me indicated he has seen this pattern in all HE patients he has treated, though a few of the HE patients I've interacted with indicated this had not been true for them personally. When I was first in the hospital, though, my knee reflexes tested as normal (2+) or once possibly slightly depressed (1-2+). There is speculation that it might have been the influence of the high thyroid antibodies, or perhaps it was too early in the illness for the knee reflexes to have changed – I'll never know for sure. When things were not going well, testing my reflexes often triggered bouts of myoclonus.

2. Cognitive Issues

a. 'Blank Brain' – This is one of the scariest symptoms for me. I have always had a very busy brain, overflowing with thoughts and emotions to the point where it was difficult to get to sleep. During this illness, my brain was very often blank, with no words, thoughts, or reactions present for hours at a time. Occasionally there would be a thought or feeling that wanted to bubble to the surface. With a lot of effort I might be able to haul it up, but a lot of the time I didn't have the energy – so it went away and my mind stayed blank. Getting a train of thought going was like trying to get a hundred-car freight train going. Once a train of thought was in motion, sometimes I could sustain it for a little while. But if the momentum stopped, it was back to square one.

b. Flat Emotions – I'd always been a very emotive person – a poetry writing major with save-the-world magnets all over my car. Given how stressful this experience could have been, it was merciful in a way that my emotions became so muted as the illness progressed. Someone told me this is called 'emotional blunting'. I had almost no feelings about my illness – even when I thought I would soon be in a nursing home, slipping from dementia into death. Day to day, I didn't laugh or make facial expressions. Even if I understood a joke and thought it was funny, nothing would happen. That was difficult for my husband, and it created a lot of distance in little ways. For example, watching a DVD was one of very few things we could still do together, but for him it was like watching a movie with a mannequin. Even when I tried to explain to him what was happening, he thought I hated everything because I didn't react at all.

c. Word-finding Troubles – I had a lot of difficulty finding ordinary words, and sometimes retrieved the wrong one. The process of converting my thoughts into words was much slower, and it took a lot more effort. Very often it felt like I was actually translating to get the words out – like when I try to speak my rusty French to someone.

d. Slowed Thinking and Reaction Times – To be less of a burden and any kind of useful, I tried for a little while to resume driving my husband the six blocks to the train, or taking myself the less-than-two-mile trek to doctor's appointments using side streets. The honking, screaming, staring and one-fingered salutes should have clued me in that this was not a good idea, but it was actually the repeated near collisions that made me stop driving. I had a lot of trouble (and made a number of scary mistakes) trying to time the spaces between cars to pull out into traffic safely, and I drove through a stop sign right in front of the police station because I got confused by all the cars and people. Slow processing and reaction times didn't just show up behind the wheel. When things were bad I couldn't follow the plot in a movie even though I'd seen it before, because I couldn't process what was happening fast enough. I had to ask my husband to repeat himself a lot. Often when people would ask me a question (especially if it was anything even mildly unexpected), nothing would happen between my ears. I heard the question. But no response at all would appear in my head, and all I could do was look at that person blankly – even if they waited a long time for me to respond. This still happens occasionally.

e. **Difficulty Concentrating** – This was one of my worst areas on my neuropsych testing, and it showed up everywhere in my life. I've always been a bit of an 'absentminded professor', but this was something else entirely. I think a major lapse in attention is how I ended up outside in my underwear (because I knew to come inside as soon as I noticed). Attention lapses resulted in safety issues like me walking out into traffic and having to be snatched from in front of unnoticed fast-moving cars. I think the attention issues were also why I couldn't really read or follow a conversation. I used to be able to read complex and unfamiliar material once and recall it in detail, but when I got sick I would lose the thread quickly and couldn't get words to string together to make meaning. I'd forget what I was saying in the middle of saying it, more often than I'd be able to finish a thought. This made it horribly difficult to write anything, which in those days was mostly an email to a doctor. It was so hard to hold more than about eight words in my head at a time, so trying to string together multiple sentences was next to impossible. I kept re-reading my own short emails dozens of times trying to get them to hang together in my mind. When things were bad, I had to ask for help from my family. This was incredibly frustrating, as before the illness I had always been able to communicate – I'd obtained an undergraduate and graduate degree in writing, was an award-winning competitive public speaker when I was younger and professional public speaker as an adult, and had been an analytical writer and executive-level presenter as a career. And now it was a struggle to make a sentence.

f. Math Problems – A silly example: I attempted to color my hair one day, and I couldn't figure out how many minutes were left until I could take the dye off. Fortunately, my husband came home and was able to tell me, though he looked at me strangely. As a child, I learned how to do math using Cuisenaire rods, and numbers have always fit together like puzzle pieces for me. In the past that allowed me to add up long strings of numbers in my head. But not anymore. While things have improved, I still generally have to use a calculator if

I'm working with more than two numbers. I don't know if this relates to those brief early troubles I had reading a clock or a map, or if those are in a category of their own.

g. 'Memory Problems' – I never experienced the full-scale amnesia that some patients do. For me, 'memory problems' were just things like trying to let the dog in twice in five minutes and panicking when I couldn't find him in the yard. Or asking my mom for Tylenol within three minutes of swallowing the Tylenol she had already given me. These situations actually turned out to be the result of the attention / concentration problems rather than true memory problems – my brain wasn't paying enough attention to record what had just happened. Nowadays I use a variety of tricks I learned from the cognitive rehabilitation therapist to get my brain to actively record memories, and I still write down anything I *need* to remember.

h. Confusion – This took many forms. Being confronted with complexity or surprise generally made my brain freeze up, and I got overstimulated and mentally paralyzed regularly. I couldn't react to a question (like 'can you feed the dog?') while doing a simple task like making tea. My brain would just stop and I could do neither, and someone would actually have to walk me through how to get back in gear. I needed help from my family setting one or two simple priorities for the day. I had to mark the day's tasks with a highlighter, and cut the 'done' items out of the list rather than scratch them out because my brain would short circuit if the page was too busy. I would try to use my brain for ordinary things and it would fail. Not long after I got out of the hospital, I went to a small church service. Walking back from the front of the room, I couldn't figure out how to get back to my chair even though there were only about thirty chairs in the place. I ended up freaking out a little and crashing through the rows like a panicked buffalo in front of a room full of strangers. Once when I went to use the microwave at home, I got confused and then punched in the unlock code for my phone and waited for something to happen. Another time, I reheated some leftovers, and then stared at them for a long time because I hadn't the faintest idea how to tell if they were 'done'. Eventually I just mutely shoved them at a confused houseguest and stared at him.

i. **Hallucinations When Transitioning Out of Sleep** – When I was in my sleeping-all-the-time phase, I would sometimes 'hear things' that were so convincing I would try to interact with them. I'd check my phone, ask who was calling my name, or be really confused why there was a personalized Allstate commercial emanating from under my pillow. Someone told me these are called hypnagogic hallucinations. I do not have them when I am well.

j. **Lost Social Awareness** – I lost my ability to pick up on basic social cues and 'read between the lines'. In a pressure cooker work environment this was one of the primary reasons my job was in jeopardy even before I became too ill to work at all. It led to major misunderstandings and had real business consequences in the boardroom. It made people angry and hostile with me and eroded my credibility, which made it even harder to get business results. People believed I was either stupid and incompetent, or insensitive and reckless. Or all of the above. Since I'd previously behaved differently, they were inclined to believe that I was doing it on purpose and insisted I could do better if I just tried. So when additional problems started to emerge – trouble reading, producing documents, or answering questions – people were already predisposed to view these issues as willful, no matter what I said to the contrary. By far the most painful impact of the loss of social awareness, though, was in the relationship with my husband. It wasn't until the cognitive rehabilitation therapist interviewed him that I learned how disregarded and lonely he felt, because I seemed to care so little about his feelings. We had no idea this was part of the illness, and I didn't even realize it was happening. It broke my heart when he said this was the hardest part of all for him – worse than taking care of all the domestic responsibilities and driving, generating all the income, and taking care of me and the dog. It was coming home to an unresponsive shell that didn't seem to care about him at all.

3. Stamina Issues

a. Easily Exhausted – Early on, cutting up a vegetable or unloading half a rack of the dishwasher would exhaust me to the point where I had to sit down on the kitchen floor and catch my breath. When I took a shower, my heart would be pounding, my pulse would race, and I would be shaking, weak and sweating, even though I used relatively cool water. I'd end up crumpled on the shower floor, and I generally had to lie down for a while afterwards to recover. My stamina for mental exertion was just about as limited.

b. Intense Fatigue and Excessive Sleep – Early on, I'd sleep over 20 hours a day. With recent research revealing that the purpose of sleep is to 'clean' your brain, I guess it makes sense that a brain under attack would have a lot of extra cleaning to do! Several months into my illness, I started tracking my sleep using a smartphone app. The average number of hours asleep each month has steadily dropped. I still have more fatigue than I'd like, and need more sleep than my husband does, but there is no comparison.

4. Fluctuation Patterns

a. Symptom Flares – My HE symptoms tend to flare if I have an intense period of sustained stress (like transitioning back to work) or am fighting a 'bug' (presumably because that stimulates my immune system and increases the antibodies?). I have Hashimoto's Thyroiditis as well as Hashimoto's Encephalopathy, so if something spikes my thyroid antibodies (which for me can include accidental gluten or germ exposure), my thyroid-related problems flare. This also happens if something really spikes my estrogen levels, like the in vitro fertilization treatments I underwent this year. In those instances, my TSH goes up and I experience a brief bout of things like intense bodily pain, GI problems, and bleeding mucus membranes.

b. Ability to Compensate – My brain is not quite the same as it was, and I do still have lingering deficits. On good days, I can generally compensate for them so that people who don't know me well would never know there was anything amiss. However, my ability to compensate for deficits decreases if I am overtired or stressed, especially when I need to deal with unfamiliar stimuli or questions.

5. Feelings

a. Loss of Identity – One of the toughest things about going through all of these strange and surreal experiences is that they can take away who you are. I had always been two things – 'smart' and 'nice'. With HE, suddenly I was neither, and with such a blank brain it was often like I didn't even exist.

b. Uncertainty – At first it's the uncertainty about what's happening and how far it will go, and whether we will ever get help. But even after diagnosis and treatment, there are so many things we'll never know. Are the minor findings on my MRI from HE or migraines? Or both? Or something else entirely? Do they signal some broader inflammatory process too microscopic to show up on an MRI? Or are they maybe just a coincidence and nothing to do with my symptoms at all? Can I really stop further damage? Can my brain repair itself? Generally the only thing that distinguishes HE from other possible causes for our symptoms is response to immunotherapy. Even if we're lucky enough to get diagnosis and successful treatment, we don't know what kind of antibody is attacking us, or which exact cell structure it's interfering with, or what it could choose to attack next. And what's really happening in our brains? Is it inflammation that's slowing things down, like snow on a highway? Or is it dead neurons our brains have to route around like traffic detours? Is there another medicine or supplement that would help us get or stay well – and on and on and on. Even with all this science, there are still no definitive answers.

c. **Stigma, Shame, and Loneliness** – The people in our lives can see some of the things that HE has brought – like myoclonus or falls – and readily understand these probably have a medical cause. But so much of what changes with HE doesn't have an overt physical sign or lab test to confirm that it's medical and not just laziness or bad character. Even just sleeping so much and failing to tune in to social cues can foster a lot of resentment, especially if you don't 'look sick'. This can create a lot of personal shame because you don't understand why you can't do what you used to do, and why you can't 'snap out of it'. We also need so much assistance – from driving us to the doctor to pulling us out of traffic when we don't notice what's going on around us. And we can't even contribute what we used to in order to make up for the extra burden that we bring. All of this can be very lonely and shaming.

d. **Fear** – For me, fear paradoxically only comes into play when I'm well enough to worry about getting sick again. What if the next flare is worse? What if it happens when I'm at work, or alone and far from home? What if next time I don't recover? How much can my husband and family take? There are no answers to these questions.

e. Losing My Voice – The difficulty and isolation of HE are compounded by the fact that our brains may not be working well enough to put things into words. Much of the time it's easier to say nothing than to try to tell others what we're going through. But it is so disempowering when your world is upside down and you can't connect with anyone. Inability to put our strange and awful experiences into words also generally means no one has any idea what we're going through. Over the months of this illness, I've tried to come up with a few analogies to help my family understand what was happening:

- ***Scuba Suit***: Sometimes I tell people it's like trying to walk in all my scuba gear (about 80 pounds) and fins. Yes, technically, I can walk. But it takes way more time, effort, and concentration than it did before I got sick. And it seems like the only thing neurologists test is whether I can take three steps in all that gear (i.e. follow their finger with my eyes, or squeeze their hand, or write four words...). They ignore how absurd it is to expect someone to function normally for the rest of their life in a scuba suit, lugging around 80 unwieldy extra pounds.
- ***Swiss Cheese***: One of the other analogies I've used is that it's like looking at the world through a piece of

cartoon Swiss cheese. You only get pieces of things, which makes everything confusing and hard to work with. There's not a lot of rhyme or reason to where the holes are (and it changes...). It's hard for people (including me!) to understand that just because one part of me works, that doesn't mean others will. Or that if something worked yesterday, it doesn't mean that it will work again today. I can't predict what will be missing, and I have to do a lot of 'filling in gaps' and compensating, so things take more time and effort – if they're possible at all.

- ***Hard Drive***: Another analogy is that my mind is like a partly-damaged hard drive. If the file I'm trying to use is written in a damaged sector, I may be able to access a little of the file, or none at all. To do the job of being me, I have to access lots of files all day long. Every time I try to do something I'm never sure whether I'm going to get an error message instead of what I want.
- ***Movie Screen***: Another image that pops into my head when trying to explain to someone what 'blank brain' is like (because it is *not* the Zenned-out state people try to cultivate in meditation): I feel like I'm sitting in an empty movie theater looking at a blank screen. My brain used to run a constant 'movie' of thoughts and feelings, and a few rows back some part of me (let's call it 'Awareness') would watch it and decide what to take

action on. Awareness still shows up when I'm awake, but I can't get the movie started. Without some kind of thought or feeling up on the screen, nothing happens. In such mental silence, there's no initiating action, planning or problem solving – even when I am awake and there are critical things that need to be done. I just sit there like computer without an operating system – powered on and totally useless.

- ***Intoxication***: If all else fails, people can usually imagine going through life drunk and sleep-deprived. With enough effort they could write an email or make a phone call, and their MRI would be normal, but you wouldn't expect them to keep their job or driver's license for very long.

Looking Forward

Getting my migraines and thyroid condition properly managed has made a huge difference in my quality of life, and other lifestyle changes like the daily fruit-and-vegetable 'super-smoothies' have had a big impact as well. The first few days on prednisone were euphoric, and after that things gradually settled into what I hope will be my 'new normal'. Outside of recognizable symptom flares, I can generally hide my residual cognitive issues from people who don't know me very well – especially with the tips and tricks from cognitive rehab. I feel incredibly lucky.

I'm able to drive safely again, though sometimes I still take a bit of extra time to find a big enough gap to pull safely into traffic. I keep a set of yellow reflective 'STUDENT DRIVER' magnets in my trunk. Primarily I used them when I was transitioning back into driving, but I can still put them on if I'm tired or on unfamiliar turf. I haven't used them in a while, but people definitely became kinder and more patient on the road when I did, and that made driving much less stressful.

Even on steroids, I have sometimes gotten symptom flares if I'm fighting a bug or I push myself too hard. For example, in the third week of my gradual transition back to work, I relapsed for a few days. I'm not sure what the long-term outcome would have been, as a few days later I got swept up in a large round of layoffs and I haven't found new work yet. It's a bit unnerving, as I know there will be a potential for relapse when transitioning into whatever job I find next, and I don't really know what a 'safe' threshold of stress and work hours would be. I do know that I will always need to be really cautious about germs, gluten, and stress, and need to keep learning newer and better ways to live with HE. We'll see what the future holds.

What I've Learned – For Patients and Caregivers

Over the last year, I've interacted with dozens of people around the world being treated for HE. In the process, a few of the most important things I've learned:

1. Autoimmune encephalopathies are far more common than generally suspected, and often misdiagnosed.
2. Getting a diagnosis can be a very long and difficult process – especially in 'milder' cases.
3. Response to immunotherapy can be all that differentiates HE from other possible diagnoses.
4. As with other autoimmune illnesses, HE is generally a persistent consideration rather than being 'cured' after a single intervention.
5. Being an informed and proactive patient or caregiver can make all the difference.

If I could give patients and caregivers some advice on this journey, it would be:

1. **Get a Frontal Assessment Battery – Early:** Frontal lobe dysfunction is hard for a stranger to pick up in a 20 minute office visit, but can wreak tremendous havoc in the real world. It's a common manifestation in HE, and it can cause us to come across as inconsiderate hypochondriacs – making it seem reasonable to minimize many of our complaints. In my case, family, co-workers, and I all initially passed moral judgment on me for things we later learned were caused by frontal lobe difficulties. Frontal lobe dysfunction can be detected by a series of simple tests called a Frontal Assessment Battery, and clinical findings early on can make a big difference in the path taken to diagnosis and treatment. If your doctor doesn't know what a Frontal Assessment Battery is, you can google it and bring the printout.

2. **You May Have to Manage Your Own Case**: In the hospital, someone different did the rounds every day. I saw a lot of busy doctors both in and out of the hospital, and none of them really communicated with each other. This meant everyone had an incomplete picture of what was happening, and it upped the odds of something getting lost in translation – like discharging me from the hospital before the thyroid antibody test results were in. Everyone thought surely someone else was coordinating my care, and they all wanted to defer to someone with more HE experience. No one would drive the bus until we found that experienced doctor – and that took months. For the best possible outcome, most of us will need to be more involved in managing HE than we ever imagined a lay person could be. If you find yourself in this situation, try to find a balance of patience and persistence. Ask questions. Give treatments time to work, but speak up if they don't. Make sure you always know what and when the 'next step' is – and follow up on the paperwork. Help others understand your 'new normal' so that they can adapt to it. All of this can be done most powerfully if you are well informed about your situation, your options, and your plan.

3. **Knowledge Is Power**: Even if you're lucky enough to get someone willing to take the lead on your case, your peace of mind and prognosis will be much better if you (whether the 'you' reading this is the patient or the primary caregiver) become as informed as possible. It can start with getting a full copy

of all records from each test and doctor visit, reading them, and looking things up online till you understand what they do and don't mean. Keep all the records together in a folder or binder, and bring them to the first appointment with any new doctor. It can also help to create an easily-skimmed spreadsheet with all the lab results in it for quick reference when a doctor asks questions. Take advantage of the HESA website and other online communities for information and support. And find a way to capture a record of how you're doing over time. Since my symptoms wax and wane, I have to track things daily in order to see patterns. Fortunately, 'there's an app for that'. I use my smartphone to track everything from symptoms to sleep – Symple for symptoms and triggers, Sleep Cycle for sleep, and My Days for weight and other info. This helps me see what makes a difference in how I feel, and to forecast what my health will allow me to do in different situations. It's what helped me figure out that even a tiny amount of gluten aggravates my thyroid problems, and it lets me tell my doctor things like "I've been sleeping 17 hours a day for the last six weeks" rather than "I'm really tired."

4. **Bring a Friend**: Especially early in your illness, it can be invaluable to bring a calm, healthy friend or family member to your appointments to ask and answer questions, and understand and remember the doctor's answers. Someone else may also be in a better position to observe and describe what's changed for you if HE has started to affect your brain. And

someone else's assertion that you're 'not yourself' may carry more weight with a new doctor than your own.

5. **Get Some Support**: Encephalopathy is a rare and poorly understood condition, and even many experienced doctors do not have sufficient experience with it to tell you what to expect, or to feel confident designing a treatment plan and long-term maintenance. For insight, information, and support, the online communities on Facebook and Inspire.com have been my lifeline, and the HESA website has been an invaluable source of scientific info. During this illness I also needed in-person help getting to doctor's appointments, dealing with all the paperwork, and many other things. Even if you have the I-can-do-it-myself gene, allow for the possibility that your self-awareness and judgment might not be as sound as you're used to, and invite and allow others to help you.

6. **Slow Down**: One of the most useful things my cognitive rehabilitation therapist taught me is the example of the struggling swimmer. In lifeguarding classes, instructors teach that frightened swimmers often do things that seem intuitive, but don't help: they struggle to keep as much of themselves out of the water as possible, and they end up exhausting themselves and going under. In the process, they can also take down anyone trying to help them. Struggling swimmers have a much better chance of reaching the shore if instead they sight their goal on the horizon, take a deep breath and relax, and swim under the surface for a little while. HE can be a bit like this. We can burn

a lot of energy reacting to our limitations – being angry, scared, or embarrassed, or 'trying harder'. Sometimes we even struggle against anyone trying to help us. Whenever we feel like we're drowning (because we're having trouble walking, or speaking, or remembering, or reacting), we can take a deep breath, calm down, and try to focus on our real goal. Swimming beneath the surface might mean letting go of our frustration and finding a different way to get something done – like using a different word than the one we wanted, rather than fighting to get the one we can't find. It can also mean allowing someone to help. The important thing is to slow down and release the struggle. We're all better swimmers when we're not in a state of panic.

7. **Remember That Doctors Are Human**: While all the doctors I've seen have had extensive training and experience, they have a short time to review massive amounts of incomplete data and vague symptoms, and may first zero in on patterns with which they have the most experience. Unless you get really lucky, HE may not be that 'comfortable old shoe' diagnosis for your doctor. You may need to bring them some scientific info to help them understand why you think this is what's happening – and recognize when it's time to look for a new doctor. My best outcomes have been with folks who specialize in one of my primary need areas – whether it's chronic migraine or cognitive rehabilitation. This isn't the same thing as shopping around until I find someone who agrees with me – I keep looking until I find someone who can help me. For example,

the initial neuropsychologist I saw focused on psychotherapy, and unsurprisingly this is the arena in which his diagnosis and treatment ideas showed up. He believed that, rather than any health problems at all, I had PTSD and mood disorders, and my problems at work were the result of a power struggle with authority figures. His prescription was biofeedback and psychotherapy. He became angry and sarcastic when I expressed doubts about this interpretation. I took the same test results to a neuropsychologist that specializes in cognitive rehabilitation, and he instantly saw the frontal lobe deficits and how they translated into the problems I was having in work and relationships, and offered strategies that produced immediate results.

8. **'Normal' Is Subjective**: Generally whatever conclusions a new specialist is going to draw about me will be based on the 20 minutes I'm in their office, and they will compare those observations with 'statistical normal'. If you used to be smarter than the average bear, or faster, or stronger, it's going to be tough to get a stranger to believe that 'age-appropriate' is a danger sign for you. Many of us who have been successfully treated were initially told our problems were everything from 'normal aging' to depression, stress, or lack of exercise. And that doesn't even count all the official misdiagnoses. The folks who have had the hardest time getting a diagnosis in 'milder' cases of HE have been those that previously had high cognitive capabilities. The U of C endocrinologist said they see this all the time with dementia patients – that it's really hard to get a

complaint of cognitive difficulty taken seriously if the patient started with a very high IQ, because the patient can fall so far before striking strangers as abnormal in a short conversation. A word of caution on this one: people can get really weird about it. A number of us have experienced some surprisingly sarcastic and condescending responses from clinicians when suggesting that 'statistical normal' is not 'our normal'. For example, the clinical psychologist who did my initial neuropsych evaluation actually waved his hands over his head and shouted at me that I must think I'm soooo much better than everyone else if normal wasn't good enough for me. It didn't matter that there was a verifiable 40+ point drop in IQ, and that some of the frontal lobe centric test results ranged in the 5th to the 18th percentiles. A number of other patients have reported similar experiences with other clinicians in other cities. I'm not sure what to attribute this to, but can only suggest treading cautiously?

9. **Get Professional Help with Disability Paperwork**: The denial of my disability insurance claim was the third of the three times I cried during this illness. The entire year I was on medical leave was without pay, because of how the paperwork was handled. If you need to go on medical leave from your job, please get expert help with the paperwork – even if you don't think you need it.

10. **HE Isn't the Only Rock to Look Under**: When dealing with a new and scary illness, it can be easy to forget that HE isn't the only thing affecting my wellbeing. On my journey to

wellness, I also need to make sure any other health conditions (like my migraines and thyroid disease) are managed well. And I need to invest energy in healthy lifestyle choices – limiting germ exposure and stress, and getting healthy sleep, food, and exercise. For me, cognitive rehabilitation also made a big difference in my quality of life, and tips and techniques designed for ADHD sufferers are helping me compensate for some of my ongoing frontal lobe problems. Even if each of these things only makes a 3% improvement in my quality of life, together they add up to a big difference. And big benefits can come from unexpected places. For example, the biggest boost to my poor beleaguered energy levels came when I started putting a pound and a half of fruit and veggies into a Vitamix blender every morning and drinking a super-smoothie. As a bonus, the super-smoothies also helped my husband deal with the stress of being an HE caregiver. Instead of just thinking about our illness, we can benefit from spending time on our wellness.

What I've Learned – For Clinicians

Conversations with other patients and caregivers have highlighted a number of issues that continue to make diagnosis particularly challenging, and I wanted to share learnings that might make things easier for physicians in the future.

1. **Spectrum of Severity**: As severe cases have received the most attention, many physicians are not aware that autoimmune

encephalopathy also has milder forms, without coma or psychosis. For many patients, years of milder symptoms precede diagnosis (and diagnosis often does not occur until after a crisis resulting in hospitalization). However, even milder forms and stages can have severe employment, relationship, and personal safety consequences due to changes in brain function, and can be helped tremendously via immunotherapy.

2. **Prevalence**: Many doctors believe autoimmune encephalopathies are rarer than they turn out to be, which often leads to dismissal of potential autoimmune causes for cognitive and neurological problems. At the November 2012 FACES conference held by Encephalitis Global, Dr. Carol Glaser of the California Encephalitis Project (CEP) indicated that of the thousands of cases CEP reviewed, a surprisingly large portion turned out to be autoimmune. Our unaffiliated 'Hashimoto's Encephalopathy' Facebook network includes SREAT patients in active treatment on five continents.

3. **Symptom Variability**: As with all autoimmune illnesses, symptom intensity can wax and wane. As with other dementias, incidents in the same timeframe can range from normal to mildly odd to alarming. A great deal of the real-world impairment in 'milder' cases of autoimmune encephalopathy comes from this inconsistency in capabilities (as well as the intense fatigue). HE also often causes attention and concentration problems, which can cause further variability in performance. Fluctuating impairment levels can complicate diagnosis if

clinicians are expecting patients to demonstrate only stable or progressive symptoms.

4. **Impairment Variability**: As with other dementias, not all areas of the brain are affected equally by autoimmune encephalopathy. For example, my neuropsych test results indicated my non-verbal problem solving skills and vocabulary remained in the 97th percentile, and I could sound coherent when discussing my symptoms. However, at the same time I would walk out of the house in my underwear without realizing it, and couldn't figure out how to navigate around a parked car when attempting to drive.

5. **Frontal Lobe Deficits**: Frontal lobe impairments are very common HE manifestations, and notoriously difficult to pin down – especially in a brief office visit with a stranger. In HE, frontal lobe impacts often include significant deficits in attention and concentration, personality changes, altered judgment, motor difficulties, speech production problems, and other changes. Impaired social and emotional functions can be sufficient to lead to job loss – especially when a medical cause is not suspected. Lapses in attention and environmental awareness can be severe enough to cause personal safety problems and gaps in memory. In patients with milder cases of HE, the deficits may not be apparent to a stranger during a typical neurological exam.

It could be tremendously helpful if initial screening for patients complaining of cognitive problems included a Frontal

Assessment Battery – a series of simple tests that can be completed in a few minutes without any special equipment or waiting for lab results. This could be combined with asking patients (or someone who knows them well) about specific examples of changes typical of frontal lobe impairment. While existence of frontal lobe issues would not confirm a diagnosis, it could help justify further investigation if other neurological tests are normal.

6. **Relative Loss**: A significant decline in cognitive performance can cause major job and relationship difficulties, even if associated neuropsych test scores are remain in the statistically normal range. This is especially true for patients starting with a high level of cognitive functioning, who can sustain significant losses without dropping outside statistical normal on neuropsych tests.

As an example, my neuropsych results showed changes such as a loss of almost 50 percentile points in verbal reasoning and over 40 IQ points relative to historical scores, but I still fell into the statistical 'normal' range for both. In the time leading up to my first hospitalization, I found my work performance radically altered, and in the absence of a medical explanation, others observing the decline often attributed it to being willfully careless or inconsiderate, saying things like "*I know you're smarter than that!*" or "*I don't know what your problem is lately but…*"

In addition to assessing cognitive capabilities relative to 'statistical normal', looking at cognitive capabilities relative to 'personal historical normal' could be diagnostically revealing. In the absence of formal 'pre-illness' neuropsych test results for comparison, perhaps patients' current capabilities could be contrasted with their historical performance on comparable standardized academic tests to illuminate potential areas of significant decline for further investigation. Soliciting observations from someone who knew the patient well before and after illness onset could also be illuminating.

7. **'Real World' Impairment**: For many reasons, performance on neuropsych tests does not necessarily correlate to performance in 'real world' activities. Relative losses and symptom variability can have serious consequences even if neuropsych and neurological test scores are not alarmingly low. For example, changes in my environmental awareness and reaction times caused me go from a driver with no traffic accidents or moving violations, to one with frequent and alarming near-collisions, who was ultimately instructed to give up driving.

8. **Impact of Emotional State**: Patients are generally pretty frightened and frustrated by the time multiple specialists are consulted, and in some cases paranoia can be a manifestation of the illness. Patients' state of agitation and compromised emotional self-regulation can encourage doctors to suspect psychogenic origins, rather than an organic cause.

9. **Impact of Complex Health Histories**: As HE generally only emerges in a context of myriad pre-existing health problems – many incompletely managed – patients can be perceived as

simple hypochondriacs due to the diversity and fluctuations of their symptoms. Patients also don't know what information in these complex health histories is relevant to diagnosis, and may therefore ramble or leave out important information. Patients also often lack a framework to articulate exactly what's changed, and we may misattribute some of our symptoms – for example citing memory problems for events missing from our memories when in fact attention problems are to blame. Symptoms of one illness can also impact those of another, and it can be very difficult to isolate cause and effect.

10. **Coordination of Care**: Autoimmune encephalopathy crosses many specialties, and without a 'case manager', the road to diagnosis and treatment can be disjointed with long delays between waypoints. It can also be difficult to get anyone to evaluate the whole picture. In my case, over two dozen doctors were involved, with almost no direct interaction among any of them.

Physicians willing to talk to other doctors can make a big difference in patient outcomes – even if they can't personally make the diagnosis or design treatment. Patients in our group who have had a physician willing to coordinate their care often had much faster times to diagnosis and better outcomes – even if the coordinating physician had no prior knowledge of or experience with autoimmune encephalopathy.

11. **Availability of Specialists**: The types of specialists generally involved in HE diagnosis are in high demand and often have

long wait times and short time slots to assess diverse patients – which can mean that data crucial to definitive diagnosis can take many months to obtain. For example, my neuropsych testing was authorized in October, and I did not receive the results until March.

If there are multiple options for screening for particular types of issues, physicians can do patients a great kindness when recommending next steps by taking into consideration how long it will likely take to get answers. For example, physicians could use tools such as the Frontal Assessment Battery early in the process to guide further investigation, rather than waiting until formal neuropsych testing results are available. Also, any assistance in coordinating communication and transitions among specialists can go a long way in speeding up access to treatment.

12. **Symptom Overlap**: Typical autoimmune encephalopathy symptoms (such as fatigue, headache, myoclonus, cognitive and personality changes, balance and coordination changes, eye problems, hallucinations, slurred speech, word finding difficulties, etc.) aren't unique to this illness, and many of the usual preliminary tests (MRI, EEG, basic neurological exam, MMSE, spinal tap, etc.) can be within normal limits across a variety of the possible diagnoses. Autoimmune encephalopathy symptoms can mirror those of more common illnesses, with steroid responsiveness (or impact of plasmapheresis, IVIG, or immunosuppressants) being the only definitive differentiator.

Many patients are initially misdiagnosed, and treated for conversion disorder, movement disorders, ataxia, complicated migraine, mood disorders, 'stress', or various forms of mental illness without improvement in symptoms. Carrying numerous diagnoses while complaining the treatments aren't helping can increase the likelihood of patients being perceived as hypochondriacs. The misdiagnoses can also be accompanied by medications with serious side effects.

If steroids or other immunotherapies are considered only as a last resort, this can result in very long wait times for help. Antibody tests early in the diagnostic process could help differentiate among the possible causes – regardless of whether autoimmunity is yet suspected. Many HE patients can have significant thyroid antibodies (showing an overall autoimmune predisposition) without showing significantly elevated TSH. In some cases, perhaps response to a short trial of immunotherapy could be used to help establish diagnosis, rather than only once diagnosis is confirmed.

Even once diagnosis is achieved, management presents ongoing challenges. Information regarding this illness is relatively new, and doctors and patients alike aren't always certain what to expect.

13. **Treatment Duration:** Many patients and doctors have been led to believe that tapering down through a single course of steroids will 'cure' them of their symptoms. However, interaction with dozens of other autoimmune encephalopathy

patients around the world has shown that, as with other autoimmune diseases, many patients do not achieve permanent remission via a single course of steroids. Though some patients have achieved extended remission via plasmapheresis and/or IVIG, such treatments can be difficult to access. To keep symptoms at bay, many patients must remain on a low to moderate steroid dose long term, or transition from steroids to immune suppressants.

14. **Treatment Effectiveness:** Immunotherapy may halt progression of the illness without fully reversing all symptoms, and as with other autoimmune conditions, overextension, stress, and activation of the immune system can still cause an upsurge in symptoms and reduced ability to compensate. Patients' symptoms can also be influenced by interplay among the other diagnoses, medications, and medicated misdiagnoses in their complex health profiles. For many patients, it can be difficult to ensure any autoimmune thyroid condition is 'completely managed', especially where treating physicians and the labs on which they rely are not aware of the clinical practice guidelines published by the American Association of Clinical Endocrinologists and the American Thyroid Association.

Doctors can help patients understand that a multifaceted and incremental approach to treatment may be required to ensure each condition is fully managed. This could require treating one condition completely and waiting to see what symptoms remain before moving to the next. When patients arrive with diagnoses and medications that may have resulted from misattribution of symptoms – especially psychiatric and movement disorders that started concurrent with autoimmune symptoms – doctors can consider whether it may be appropriate to coordinate with other physicians to determine whether HE might be a better explanation for the patient's symptoms, and if so whether adjustment to the patient's other diagnoses and treatments may be appropriate. Doctors can also work with the patient's other physicians to make sure comorbid conditions are fully managed, and can encourage patients to join HESA and other organizations for support and information about HE and associated treatment strategies.

15. **Cognitive Rehabilitation**: Even once a 'flare' has been quieted, most patients have residual cognitive changes. With extra effort, many patients can compensate for some of these changes as long as they are otherwise healthy and well-rested. Cognitive rehabilitation can help with adaptive strategies for when symptoms are more active, or when stress and fatigue overwhelm natural ability to compensate. An experienced cognitive rehabilitation therapist can also help patients understand exactly how their capabilities have changed, how to gauge 'how they're doing' if their self-awareness is compromised, and how to manage risks and commitments as their capabilities fluctuate. As an example, those whose frontal lobes are impacted by HE may be able to benefit from many of the same compensating strategies used to assist those with ADHD. Physicians could make a

world of difference for patients by identifying and referring to cognitive rehabilitation therapists who can help patients adapt to their dynamic 'new normal'.

Finally

I hope that the stories in this book help patients to know they are not alone, and that the information in these pages assists readers on the quest for understanding and wellness. For all the HE patients out there: I'm sorry you're going through this, and I wish you the very best!

Lisa F (age at diagnosis: 38)

I will begin my story with the fact that autoimmune diseases run in my family, including Polymyositis, Sjogren's Syndrome, Hashimoto's Thyroiditis, Antiphospholipid Syndrome, Hypokalemic Periodic Paralysis, Pernicious Anemia, Fibromyalgia, Rheumatoid Arthritis, Narcolepsy and Raynaud's Disease. When my mom and I would watch episodes of Mystery Diagnosis, it seemed like we always knew a family member who had one of the rare diseases or syndromes highlighted on the show!

I was diagnosed with narcolepsy at age 27, but my journey into autoimmune hell didn't start until I was 40. I first started noticing that I was always short of breath and had no energy and the muscles in my legs and arms were weak. My heart rate was very fast all of the time (usually between 90 & 120 beats per minute) and I was (and am still) constantly sweating after just a little exertion or when stressed out. I was diagnosed with Grave's Disease in March of 2011 and had radioiodine therapy to kill my thyroid in May of 2011 due to the tachycardia and weakness.

As I went from being hyperthyroid to hypothyroid over the next several months, I had to stop taking my medicines for narcolepsy as stimulants were not helping the tachycardia I was experiencing. I had to stop working for a few months until I was able to start my narcolepsy medications again. During this time, I was very tired and confused and unable to make even simple decisions. I do not remember most of this time.

In June of 2011 I went back to work. I began experiencing many new symptoms. The building I worked in was laying new carpet and it appeared that I was really sensitive to the adhesive. It seemed as though every time they laid carpet in a new area I would start feeling funny and get strange symptoms that included tachycardia; facial flushing; one eye would appear larger than the other; the left side of my face, neck, half of my tongue, arm and hand would get numb or tingly; my muscles and joints hurt; I was unable to concentrate; my time management was poor; I was unable to make even the smallest decision; things that normally took ten minutes were now taking a half hour to an hour. I had very poor short term memory and would need to read things over and over again.

I had a lot of problems with speech. I could not find the right words and would often use words that were incorrect, but somehow related to the one I intended to use. I started to stutter, which was something I had never done before. I began to have (and still have) difficulty performing arithmetic calculations. I could not remember things that were said to me verbally. I would sometimes hear, but not retain, the words people spoke. It was as if I could only comprehend the last five words, and the rest would be lost.

I was always tired and would fall asleep easily, even with medication. I couldn't read anything that was long or had too much information because I would not be able to comprehend more than a few sentences. Needless to say, my work performance was sorely lacking.

Prior to getting sick, my favorite hobbies were reading fantasy novels, doing number and logic puzzles, and researching new things. I was very creative and always coming up with new ideas and it seemed as though my mind was always active.

As time went on, I lost the motivation to do anything other than go to work, and I would be too tired to do anything else once I got home. I often fell asleep on the bus ride home. (I had given up my driver's license due to fatigue and increased severity of cataplexy - loss of muscle control during episodes of strong emotion – usually laughter – due to narcolepsy not under control). Once home I would eat dinner and go back to sleep. I spent very little time with my family and friends.

I went to my doctor several times and at first everyone thought that all of the symptoms were due to my thyroid not yet being at a normal level. I remembered how great I had felt when the endocrinologist gave me steroids prior to the radiation therapy on my thyroid. I brought this up to my doctor in January of 2012 and she said she recently had referred a patient to a neurologist, and that patient had Hashimoto's Encephalopathy. She said that since that diagnosis is so rare, she didn't think it was possible for me to have it too, but she said if I had another flare up, she would be willing to try steroid therapy.

A few months later, she left the clinic and I had to start over with a new doctor. He was fantastic and listened to everything I had to say and he agreed to start steroid therapy to see if the symptoms got any better. I started feeling great! My muscle and joint pains went away, I was not short of breath, I could walk long distances, my brain fog went away, memory improved, speech got better, I had more energy, the numbness and tingling went away, and I just felt so much better. Both my primary care doctor and neurologist agreed that a diagnosis of Hashimoto's Encephalopathy fit my symptoms as well as response to steroid therapy. Unfortunately, my blood sugar went up, I gained weight, and the doctors weaned me off the steroids.

I again started feeling poorly and I slowly started experiencing many of the same symptoms again. In late October 2012, I went to the emergency room from work due to tachycardia. My heart rate went up to 153 bpm and I felt very funny. They kept me overnight for observation, and did not find a cause. I had a stress echocardiogram and my heart was fine. I followed up with my primary physician and he agreed to refer me to the Mayo Clinic in Rochester, Minnesota due to symptoms not improving and abnormal test results.

At the Mayo clinic they found several things wrong with me, however at that time my neurological issues were in "remission". I found out I now have sleep apnea due to weight gain, I was anemic due to a large polyp in my rectum (which was removed), I was hypothyroid again and diagnosed with Hashimoto's Thyroiditis in addition to Grave's Disease. I had a few abnormal test results that were not definitive, but might point toward lupus (I had a weakly positive ANA and double stranded DNA, elevated rheumatoid factor, and elevated CRP inflammation). My MRI, EEG, EMG and spinal fluid were all normal (aside from a slightly high opening pressure in spinal fluid). My thyroid medication was increased, I started taking iron and vitamin B complex, and my narcolepsy medication was decreased.

At the present time my hemoglobin and thyroid levels are normal, my CRP inflammation is at 19.6, my narcolepsy medication has been decreased and propranolol has been increased and I no longer have tachycardia.

I use a CPAP machine while I sleep which is helping control the sleep apnea. I have some insulin resistance and blood sugar tends to run high.

My vitamin D levels have been low even though I have been taking high levels of vitamin D for over a year. I still start sweating excessively with little exertion, and am frequently tired. I will be starting occupational therapy to try to get my math and speech skills back to normal so I can get back to work. I still have problems making decisions and have word finding issues occasionally. Stress seems to make symptoms worse. I don't think I will ever be able to drive again due to cataplexy as well as inability to make decisions quickly. I am on short term disability which runs out soon.

Having Hashimoto's Encephalopathy has changed my life in many ways. I keep things very simple and try to keep stress levels down to a minimum, I sleep a lot more, I allow myself extra time to recover from outings and I try not to do anything that will wear me out. When my speech is bad and I stutter and have word finding difficulties, I try to slow down and then I laugh it off rather than get upset.

I try not to go into crowded or loud places and if I have to, I try not to stay very long. My family knows not to put me on the spot for quick answers to questions or quick solutions to problems. I am so different than I used to be. I still have very little memory of an entire year of my life. The worst part is that I don't look sick. It's hard to make people understand my limitations when I look fine to them.

Laura (age at diagnosis: 33)

First, just a bit about myself. I am a 34 year-old- female, mother of two wonderful kids, and wife to an awesome husband. I could not make it through this journey without the support of my loving and wonderful family. I am a school psychologist and work for a public school system, providing intervention, consultation, and assessment for children with learning and behavioral issues.

Looking back on my health issues, I have been sick for some time. Although these issues were not related to HE, I think they started the process which led me to HE today.

In 2005 after the birth of my first child, I developed hyperthyroidism. This was identified after presenting with fatigue, weight loss, and anxiety shortly after the birth of my daughter (8 weeks after delivery). At first, the doctor thought I was dealing with post-partum issues. However when I told him that I had a thyroid nodule that had been identified by my gynecologist at my last visit, he decided to perform additional testing. TSH levels were drawn and found to be in the hyperthyroid range, explaining my symptoms and issues. I was referred to an endocrinologist for follow-up. My endocrinologist performed additional testing and after first being diagnosed with Graves ' disease, the diagnosis changed to Hashimoto's Thyroiditis once all blood work had returned.

Over the next five years (during which I had another child in 2007), I was in a constant cycle of needing thyroid medication and not needing thyroid medication, as the disease was causing constant fluctuations in my TSH (i.e. sometimes too much and sometimes not enough). I never really felt well, rested, or healthy.

During the summer of 2010 things really seemed to level out, and I did not need thyroid medication as my levels had stabilized on their own. In the winter of 2010, something weird happened. I suddenly developed severe insomnia and anxiety. I had always suffered from mild forms of both; however this was severe. I was honestly sleeping only 2 hours a night on average. I was also severely fatigued but unable to sleep. I started getting very upset because these symptoms were out of nowhere and had no explanation.

This continued from December of 2010 until January 2011, during which time I did seek medical attention. My doctor ran all kinds of tests including thyroid levels; however all results were optimal and normal. He basically chalked it up to anxiety. I was prescribed medication for sleep which did help, and after a long 8 weeks, miraculously the issues cleared up on their own with no other medications. I am not sure if this was HE related, but I look back and wonder if this was the beginning of some issues.

Fast forward to the summer of 2011, the best summer ever! I felt great and had no issues. I still did not need or require thyroid medication. I continued feeling well until the Fall/Winter of 2011. In January of 2012, something began to change.

The first thing I noticed was severe eye issues and severe fatigue. My eyes became very fatigued, swollen, dry, etc. I did not know what this was at first and thought perhaps my thyroid was causing me issues. I started to take thyroid medication again, hoping to clear the problems. However, despite weeks of medication, the issues persisted. This continued through February, March, and April with no relief. Basic blood tests and labs continued to come back normal and doctors were mentioning things like Chronic Fatigue Syndrome, etc.

Everything changed in May. I remember bits and pieces leading up to my hospitalization but some things I still cannot remember clearly at all. Things worsened pretty rapidly. I clearly remember that Tuesday, May 1st, 2012 was a bad day. I was at work, talking with my boss and good friend. She was asking me what was wrong, and I broke down and started crying. I told her that my fatigue was debilitating, and that same day I noticed something was "off" with my balance. My thinking was also unclear and foggy (as I call it).

I remember telling her I was scared that I had Multiple Sclerosis (MS) or a brain tumor. I was scheduled to see my endocrinologist (who was two hours away) the next day. She gave me hope that maybe he could help me and answer my questions/address my problems.

That night something weird also happened with my eyes. I was in the living room reading and all of a sudden my eyes started to dart back and forth uncontrollably and would not stop. This happened several times. I remember telling my husband something weird was happening with my eyes. I googled and found out it was possibly nystagmus. When I read the causes of nystagmus, I remember becoming concerned.

The next morning when I awoke my balance was even worse. The brain fog had worsened, and I had extreme difficulty thinking and remembering things. I could remember them, but it took me a while to recollect my thoughts and memories. I felt "surreal" and for lack of a better term like "Alice in Wonderland". Things seemed off.....like looking at yourself from the outside in. I was also very light-headed, had vision issues (grainy like a black and white screen on an old television set), and felt like I was constantly on a rocking boat.

The crazy thing is....I drove myself to the appointment with my endocrinologist that day. I don't even know how I made it. I remember pulling off the road several times and picking up the phone to call my husband to come get me. However, he was at work (far away), and I felt guilty. I am a stubborn, independent person too, and I basically forced myself to make it. I look back and realize this was so dangerous!

At the appointment, the endocrinologist offered to switch my thyroid meds from Synthroid to Armour, as he said this helped some people. He also indicated that the issues I was describing were not thyroid related, and that I should check back with my primary care doctor about my symptoms. I somehow made it back home that day, collapsing into my bed around 7:00 or 8:00 at night.

The next morning (Thursday) was even worse. I woke up to get ready for work and ran into the wall. I could not think clearly or see clearly. I remember my husband asking me what was wrong, and I broke down in the bathroom crying: Something is really wrong! He told me I needed to see our doctor, and I agreed.

I called in sick that day and went to my doctor's walk-on clinic as he had no open appointments. I saw a physician assistant (P.A.) and she seemed concerned but told me it was likely my ear (i.e. vertigo). The issues with thinking were not really addressed that day by the P.A. However, she did order a MRI but indicated that it would be a few days before they could get me in the schedule.

I left that day crying and scared. Friday morning, things continued to worsen (this was the pattern). I had an OBGYN appointment that morning, and my husband had to take me (he also filled me in on all these details!). I was slurring words and speech at that point. My husband demanded help and answers from my OBGYN. When she saw me, she was so concerned that she immediately called my doctor. My primary doctor was out of town. Therefore she spoke to his colleague, and he agreed to see me right away.

At the doctor's office, he did several tests (i.e. following his finger with my eyes, asking questions). My husband said I was not making total sense and seemed very out of it. He had to physically lead me/hold onto me due to my balance issues, and they finally had to get a wheelchair to get me out of the building. The doctor was puzzled and thought I might have some weird viral inner ear issue. I guess they kept returning to this because of my balance issues. However, I did not have vertigo; it was more of a rocking/shifting feeling. Regardless, due to my issues the doctor said he wanted to cover all bases and run some additional tests.

I was then directly admitted to the hospital. My husband took me there. I have no memory of driving there, getting there, or checking in. At the hospital, they called the hospital neurologist because of my symptoms. I vaguely remember bits and pieces of the neurologist speaking to me. I remember him asking me what year it was, how many children I had, etc. I also remember him asking me my birthday, alarm code, and pin number, none of which I could recall. I remember being very scared and thinking "I am dying or have a brain tumor."

At the hospital, I was told he observed monoclonal jerking in my face and body, balance issues, nystagmus, slurred speak, and incoherent thinking. Tons of tests were ordered: blood work, EKG, EEG, MRI, and spinal tap. After getting my history and learning of my thyroid issues, my neurologist mentioned a condition called Hashimoto's Encephalopathy (HE) that had been showing up more and more in literature. He indicated that it was caused by the same antibodies that attack the thyroid. Basically, these antibodies can also attack the brain. My husband was floored!

Looking back, I am floored that he mentioned this so early. However, some of my tests had already returned normal, and I believe he was going through the process of elimination. He said I was too young to have a stroke and that the waxing and waning of symptoms along with all other issues I exhibited led him to believe this could be HE. He further explained to my husband that test results including a spinal tap will show up "normal" for many people. The only test that is consistently elevated is the Anti-TPO antibodies (thyroid antibodies). They tracked down my TPO antibody test results from years past, as I already showed positive for these but always maintained a certain baseline even from the beginning of my disease. My TPO antibodies have always hovered around 200. My results from the hospital were 1500. The neurologist believed that this surge in antibodies was the root of my problems and that this activated HE in my body. He indicated that the only true way to know if HE was the issue was to see how I responded to a high dose of IV steroids. IV steroids were begun after all other tests were completed. I was given 1000 mg a day by IV for three days.

The results were AMAZING. I began to feel better after the first treatment. However, when I say better, I mean better, but nowhere near normal or resolved. I could think more clearly and the jerking had stopped. By day three, things continued to improve. They decided to discharge me and sent me home on 60 mg of prednisone with follow-up appointments with my regular doctor and a doctor 2 hours away with HE experience.

At discharge I was feeling clearer. However, my balance issues remained. I could not walk without assistance or without holding onto walls or chairs. I was still very fatigued and an emotional wreck with the news that I had this disease that was not curable (although treatable).

At home, I slept at least 12 hours a day or more. This continued for weeks. After two weeks, I remember thinking, "This will never resolve" as I still had many of the same issues. After about eight weeks things started to calm down. My balance was better, fatigue better, but still nowhere near pre-HE.

Fast forward to today. Well, it has been almost exactly a year since my diagnosis. The last year has been trying and difficult to say the least. I have had some really good days (actually a period of 4 weeks where I felt normal) and lots of bad days. I have been to numerous doctor appointments and checkups. To be absolutely sure (at my discretion) that I did not have some weird ear issue (I was also a tad bit in a denial phase), I went to a neurotologist for balance testing, etc. He indicated that I did not have any inner ear issues but permanent damage to my balance system caused by HE in his opinion. This was just additional support of my already confirmed diagnosis. However, I needed to hear it again.

My symptoms have waxed and waned through the year. I was weaned down on prednisone, all the way to 5 mg. This process was horrible and inflammation reared its ugly head numerous times. I had a small relapse in January (triggered by a urinary tract infection) and had to be admitted to the hospital for 5 days where I received a 5-day treatment of IVIG. I am very blessed that insurance has agreed to pay for this treatment. I also currently receive an IVIG treatment on a monthly basis, and I am still on 25 mg of prednisone.

I was going to start the weaning process again but after another setback three weeks ago, I am still at 25 mg. Three weeks ago I was prescribed birth control/hormone replacement to help regulate my hormones. However, no one told me that estrogen binds to thyroid medication. This caused my TSH to increase, which resulted in an increase in my TPO antibodies, which in turn led to an increase in HE symptoms. The four weeks prior to this was when I felt "normal".

I am disheartened by the set-back. The hardest thing about this is that I don't look sick. People see me each day and assume I feel good. Of course, that is mostly my fault as I don't want people to feel sorry for me, and I don't want to be a Debbie Downer all the time. I also feel guilty saying "I feel sick" or "I feel tired" especially to my family. I feel that I am a burden to them at times.

Despite all of this, I feel so blessed. Blessed because many of the loving and caring people on the HE Facebook support group had to deal with this disease for years and years before someone diagnosed them. They have permanent damage that causes them great distress. Also, some of these same people were in a coma and much worse than me.

I know that I am lucky that it was caught so early because although I have some permanent damage, it is not as severe as others.

I am very grateful to that neurologist. Because HE was diagnosed so early, I have been able to semi-manage my symptoms and still work. Some days, however, I just have to call in because the fatigue is so bad and my thinking is fuzzy.

I worry about the future and my ability to continue to work. However I will have to take things day-by-day and deal with that when and if the time comes. My hope is that I (as well as the others) can overcome this! I have truly learned the importance of living life to the fullest and cherishing each day. Because....each day is a blessing to me and although it is hard to believe in the moment, the bad ones are blessings too! I get to be a mommy, a wife, a daughter, a co-worker, and a friend to others. Good day or bad.....I'll take it! God surely has blessed me, guided me, and helped me through this journey!

Chuck (age at diagnosis: 66)

The year 2011 was supposed to be a great year for me. My wife and I were in the process of purchasing a new home and we both were going to be officially retired. My retirement was scheduled for October 31, Halloween, and we had just hired my replacement in September.

I first began having symptoms in late September. I would be talking to someone and completely forget what I was saying as I was speaking. Everyone thought it was just me starting my retirement early and letting go, and so did I. After this had happened a few times my wife started to think maybe something was wrong, but she was not sure until the end of October, when I had to ask my son to figure out the tip after we had dinner together.

The house closed on October 28th, so we were getting ready to begin moving into our new home. I had taken a few loads to the new place and on November 3rd my wife says I went to bed and didn't get up. All I remember during this time was having a very bad ear ache in my right ear. My wife knew something was terribly wrong and had called my daughter to come help her out. This was a great decision on her part, as when moving day came, I was a complete zombie. My daughter was able to gather some of her old friends and she and my wife were able to get us moved without my help.

About a week before Thanksgiving, my wife, after having taken me to our family doctor, took me to emergency. When she did, my memory had deteriorated to a point where I could not remember the names of our four dogs. They thought I was having a stroke and admitted me for further testing. After three days and many tests, they concluded there was nothing wrong and released me.

My wife had called all of our relatives together for Thanksgiving, because I was still not responding very well. I have no memory of the holiday, other than there were people at my house. My wife's uncle told me later that I had taken him out in the backyard and tried to tell him what we were planning on doing, but could not put my sentences together very well. I do not drink, but during this time many friends and neighbors thought I was drinking because I slurred my words and my balance was off.

Three days after Thanksgiving, I was admitted to the hospital again, this time I could not even remember my wife's name. They ran some more of the same tests and some new ones, MRI's on my head, full body scans of my thorax and stomach, and they did a spinal tap. They were still having problems with a diagnosis, but the spinal tap showed it was viral, so they diagnosed me with viral encephalitis and began giving me different types of medications. One of them was Keppra, and it knocked me for a loop. Nothing was helping until they gave me some pretty strong steroids, which helped me almost immediately. The downside was I began to hallucinate, and for three days I thought the hospital was a cruise ship. To this day, I still believe sometimes I was on a ship. My wife had to take me back once to show me the hospital was not docked to a pier. I also had another hallucination where I thought I was locked in the San Leandro police department and they would not let me out. I was not in jail, they just would not let me out of the building. Later I realized it was the hospital personnel and not the police that would not let me out of the building.

When they were doing the spinal tap on me, I thought I was being held down in the shower by the male nurse and someone else. After ten days in the hospital I was released on December 8th, 2011. I was able to get through the holidays with no apparent symptoms and thought everything was OK, although my wife tells me I would get up in the middle of the night and go from room to room, like I was "mapping out" the rooms.

Because I had just changed my medical insurance, I had a very high deductible and was planning on going back to work for a short time to pay my medical expenses. Unfortunately, when my old boss called to offer me a consulting job, I was in the midst of having a relapse. I don't remember what I said, but it sure ruined my chances of working for him again.

I was admitted again to the hospital on January 16th, the day before my wife's birthday, in a semi-comatose state. Something I forgot to mention, all the time I spent in the hospital, I had someone watching me 24 hours a day because I would wander about during the hallucinations. The testing started again. I went through another round of MRI's and CT scans, but fortunately no additional spinal tap. They started giving me steroids again and I started hallucinating again. This time I was locked inside the Oakland, CA police department and I was also in a hallucination that I was involved in a massive resistance to the building of the new Eden Hospital right next door. It's funny, but my clearest remembrances of my experiences are of the hallucinations I had the last two times I was in the hospital. They were so real!

I believe it was on the third day I was in the hospital they thought they had a diagnosis as that was when they started giving me Intravenous Immunoglobulin (IVIG). I was still not given a diagnosis, but I started to settle down a little. The hallucinations were not as intense and I started feeling like myself again. I was on a regime of the IVIG for five days and was released from the hospital. This time I was put on Prednisone, 60 mg daily, Clonazepam 0.5mg to sleep and Citalopram Hydrobromide 20mg for anxiety. I had a scheduled appointment with my Neurologist a week after I was discharged and that is when I was told I had SREAT/HE. Apparently there is a test you can do with the thyroid that will tell you if it is acting up and my results were ten times higher that they should have been.

After I was discharged this last time I experienced a period of depression, anxiety and I started to have recurring nightmares. It was at this time that I changed my medical to the Veterans Administration (VA) as I had been in Vietnam. I had been diagnosed with PTSD several years before and the SREAT/HE only made it worse. At one point I was so depressed and anxious I didn't think life was going to get any better. I was told one day by a friend of mine who experienced depression that it would get better, but I didn't believe him. I was told by the psychiatrist that the Citalopram could take up to six weeks to have any impact on me, and finally one day it kicked in. It was like a huge weight had been lifted from my shoulders. I was in the 3rd week of 18 weeks of therapy when it happened and could not believe it. What a blessing.

I was kept on a 60mg a day regimen of Prednisone until May, at which time we started the dosage reduction of 5mg per month until at last I was at 0 in April of 2012. I was very fortunate in that I did not experience many of the side effects of Prednisone, although this is definitely where the nightmares started.

Since I was released from the hospital on January 24th, 2012, I had felt pretty good until I ended the Prednisone in April of 2013. Since that time my joints and muscles have ached terribly. In the morning I cannot make a fist, my back aches most of the time and I have strong pain in my shoulder along with regular pain in my joints. I tried to reduce the dosage of Citalopram down to 10mgs, but I started to experience depression and anxiety again and went back to the regular dosage.

Today I have my good days and bad days in relation to joint pain. Yesterday was sunny and warm and I had minor pain, today is cloudy and cold and I have pretty bad joint pain, especially in my shoulder. I feel fortunate in that I can still drive and work around the house and the garden. I have always been active and I thought in my retirement I would be much more productive, but at least I'm still able to do some of the things I want to do; I just do some of the work each day. I am also more conscious of my symptoms: At times if I can't remember something, or my ear starts hurting; or I get really tired, I sometimes start to panic, but soon that goes away. I'm very optimistic about life, and there is one thing that is great everyday: retirement!

I'm not a religious person, but I believe in God, and since my illness I have reestablished my communication with Him. Because of this, I have begun to fear death less and have put my life in His hands. If it is my time to go, then so be it, I must go. I do enjoy life more than I did before, because I now know how quickly it can be taken away.

Susan-Ann (age at diagnosis: 56)

Before I got sick I was a Type A personality with a Ph.D., working as a School Administrator. I had one child and was very busy with work. A few months before I became ill I was involved in organizing an international conference, which was a high stress period for me.

About a month before I was hospitalized, one evening when I could not recognize my own writing. I knew there were letters but I could not understand them. This feeling passed in a few hours.

Oct 15, 2010 was the date of my first visit to the ER. I went to work in the morning, feeling a bit out of sorts. I thought it might just be a flu bug but as I drove I realized I was not really aware of what I was doing and things got worse. I developed stroke like–symptoms: some numbness in my right arm and leg, extreme headache, dizziness, and loss of balance. I went to the ER by ambulance.

They ran some tests, including bloodwork, and my diagnosis was possible TIA.

On Oct 27, I returned to the ER, although at a different hospital, with symptoms of confusion, slurred speech, aphasia (I could understand what people were saying but when I tried to speak I had no control over the words that came out), memory loss (I didn't know where I lived or my birthdate, etc.) This time I spent a few days in the neurology ward.

While I was in the hospital I had an EEG, MRI, CT Scan, and bloodwork. Most tests came back normal, except my EEG which showed diffuse slowing on the left side, and my spinal tap which shows a high lymphocyte count. I received a possible diagnosis of "Handl" (headache, neurological deficit and lymphocytosis) or "Complicated Migraine."

In mid November I suffered ongoing migraines and my neurologist prescribed prednisone for a one week trial. I did not notice any drastic changes.

My third ER visit occurred on December 15. I was showing symptoms of psychosis. I was having hallucinations (mainly auditory), paranoia, and confusion, as well as word finding problems. I couldn't write, had difficulty with balance, and my leg muscles kept twitching. I was re-admitted to the neurology ward and most of the previous tests were repeated (EEG, CAT Scan of chest, Ultrasound, Spinal Tap, MRI, bloodwork). My TSH levels were found to be high so I was prescribed Synthroid.

I was seen by at least two neurologists, but it was someone on the endocrinology team who suggested possible Hashimoto's Encephalitis. On January 6, 2011 my neurologist "officially" gave the working diagnosis of HE and started me on 60 mg prednisone. Most major symptoms abated after 1 week.

Eighteen months after initial hospitalization I still have problems with memory, attention, and concentration. I use lots of strategies to "remember" things, such as calendars (month, week and day), and I carry a book with me to write down all phone calls I make and any information I might need to know. I have some language problems, such as word finding and spelling.

I can't filter or block out background sounds and get easily overwhelmed in noisy or busy environments. Bright lights, including sunlight, bothers me. If I have a busy day (more than one activity/appointment) I need a day to recuperate. All of these situations can result in migraines.

In terms of rehabilitation, from May to October 2011, I met weekly with an Occupational Therapist at the Acquired Brain Injury Program of a local Rehabilitation Center, who helped me understand the effects of the encephalitis and develop strategies to compensate. I have been seeing a psychologist at the center to deal with the emotional impact of my limitations. It was a real blow to my ego and major change of lifestyle. I have had to change my view of myself from helper and high achiever (working in Special Education) to being a person with a disability.

I was enrolled in an "attention group" at the center with other patients with brain injury to work on divided, sustained, selective attention skills. My GP and the staff at the center have been incredibly supportive.

In terms of medication, from March to June of 2011 I decreased prednisone until I reached 10 mg per day, which I stayed on until January 2012. The next 5 months I reduced that dose by 1 mg/month and am currently at 1 mg a day. I also take: amitriptyline, verapamil, (migraine prevention) rantidine, (ulcer prevention) synthroid, (thyroid), and alendronate (because of calcium depletion caused by prednisone)

I have not returned to work since I became ill. I am nearing retirement age and both my GP and neurologist agree that I should not return to work. Despite the damage it has done to my brain, this illness has forced me to face my mortality, learn to appreciate the little things and be thankful every day that I am alive.

Linda

As told by her daughter, Trish

My mom is Linda, and she was diagnosed with HE in 2008 by a Rheumatologist by the name of Dr. Sean Whelton at Georgetown University Hospital in Washington, D.C.

Initially at Georgetown we sought out the care of a neurologist, Dr. Carlo S. Tornatore. He ordered various diagnostic tests on my mom: MRI of the brain, basic blood tests, and an EMG. All for the complaints of extreme fatigue, and ataxia (she would be walking totally normal and without warning she would stagger to the point of almost falling). These were her reported symptoms initially, (not knowing then what we know now…that she had many more symptoms of HE but to our knowledge then, they were non-relevant to the present problem). So with these primarily two symptoms, she had sought a diagnosis on and off for about a year and a half with her local doctors.

My mom lives in a small, somewhat rural town in the Southwestern part of Virginia named Abingdon. Her local doctors failed to find anything conclusive in their assessments and diagnostics, so their conclusion was that it had to be psychological!!! To this day, after a confirmed diagnosis AND successful treatment by renowned physicians from one of the most prestigious facilities, her primary care doctor still will not recognize or believe her diagnosis of HE. Needless to say, after twenty some years he is no longer her physician.

Enter my role, my name is Trishia, I am a Registered Nurse, only child of Linda. In 2008 I was working at Georgetown University Hospital as a Clinical Administrator. I had come to know of the excellent neurology team of doctors at GUH, one of the nurse's favorites being Dr. Tornatore…for his genuine personality, smile, and caring. Not to mention being an exceptionally talented neurologist.

My mom was so exasperated by the lack of answers for her condition. At the time she was a very active 60 year old woman who enjoyed reading, going to the gym to workout, visiting family, and shopping. She was always very independent and very capable of doing anything. All of these things she enjoyed so much were coming rapidly to a halt due to the extreme fatigue and never knowing when the "imbalance" would "act up" while she was out and about in public.

She began not wanting to go out for fear of staggering suddenly and people thinking she was intoxicated or somehow purposefully debilitated. She would notice the more tired she was, the worse her imbalance would be.

Her medical history at that time was significant for hypothyroidism, GERD, degenerative joint disease, depression/anxiety, Vitamin D deficiency, Vitamin B12 deficiency, arthralgia, and migraines. She was on 100mcg of Levothyroxine, 20 mg Omeprazole, 500 of Calcium, 12.5 mg of hydrochlorothiazide for fluid retention only, 300 mg of Zantac, 180 mg of Fexofenadine HCl, 50 mg of Zoloft, daily. She received monthly B12 shots, Alprazolam 0.25 mg as needed, Ibuprofen 800 mg as needed, and Xanax 0.25 mg as needed.

I suggested she come up to Georgetown (seven hours from her home) so we could get her into see somebody that could figure this out. After getting in with Dr. Tornatore and not really learning anything concrete initially, he suggested we see Dr. Whelton, a rheumatologist, to rule out some other autoimmune diseases like Lupus.

I was eager for mom to see him. As a nurse, I've always heard that if no one can figure out what is wrong with you then go see a Rheumatologist. Wow, that saying was spot on. He ordered about twelve vials of blood (and no, I'm not exaggerating) be drawn for pages of different tests.

Within a few days as I was driving down to North Carolina he called and said "I know what's wrong with your mom, she has Hashimoto's Encephalopathy." He went on to explain about the thyroid antibodies and how hers were "off the charts high". Thus, confirming the diagnosis of HE.

Dr. Whelton went on to tell me that he and Dr. Tornatore had previously treated one other patient with HE, I later found out that person had been a speech writer for the President of the United States. So finally a diagnosis.

I was so thrilled to be able to call mom and tell her someone had finally figured it out. Now, what the heck is it and how do we make it go away forever? That was the next task at hand. Google searching back in 2008 about HE yielded little information except how rare it was, the normal protocol for IV steroid treatment and hope for remission, that was about it.

In November of 2008, they began IV methylprednisone 1000 mg monthly and methotrexate 7.5 mg weekly. By May 2009 she had experienced a nice response to the current treatment. She had marked improvement in her gait and tremor of the legs (which was a new symptom). She still had some gait instability but felt she was over 60% better. The doctors planned to continue the current treatment for another six months.

In November 2009 she had finished one full year of IV steroid plus methotrexate. She at that time felt fatigue was 40% better, however balance while walking was still not perfect. At this time she reported waking up in the middle of the night with severe lower abdominal pain along with numbness and tingling of upper extremities. These episodes reportedly lasted up to thirty minutes and would resolve spontaneously.

The neuro team decided to continue the IV steroid another six months and increase the methotrexate to 15 mg/week over the next three months to maintain an adequate level of immunosuppression.

By February 2010 my mom felt she was having a very slow but significant decline since November. Fatigue was a very significant problem however she began experiencing more tremors in the lower extremities which has interfered with her gait. She also felt her cognition was worse. On exam she had mild parasthesis in the distal lower extremities. Her tremor of the right leg looked like a resting tremor due to secondary Parkinsonism from the HE. Given the worsening of symptoms as well as the worsening fatigue and cognition, the doctor discussed the need to move on to immunosuppressive therapy stronger than methotrexate. He recommended Cytoxan infusions monthly. They stopped the methotrexate and wanted to start the Cytoxan in March, also a trial of Azilect for Parkinsonian symptoms. The dosage for Cytoxan was 720 mg (400 mg/m2), to be given with Mesna and Anzamet.

For the next month my mom attempted to have her local doctors carry out the Cytoxan infusion per Georgetown's protocol. This did not work out well. They ran the infusion too fast, didn't give the Mesna as ordered, and didn't pre/post hydrate with IV fluids. The local group's rationale: that's not the way their used to giving Cytoxan…so you disregard the physicians orders altogether?

Needless to say, that was the last time she had the infusion down there. Unfortunately for my folks, it looks like they'll have to make that seven hour road trip. Did I mention my mom doesn't really like to drive up the interstate highway? My dad brings her each time. Thanks to the wonderful people who started the HE Facebook pages and HESA – we have since learned that many years ago, maybe twenty, my mom was experiencing what may have been part of HE symptoms way back then.

My mom was driving up the interstate and passing a tractor trailer truck. She felt very anxious as the trucks often veered out of their lanes. She experienced what can only be described as an out of body like experience. She could see herself down in the car driving past the tractor trailer truck. In January 2011 her Cytoxan was held due to development of shingles. Her tremor at this point had never really improved. She now has a resting tremor of both the upper and lower right extremities. Insomnia is a problem; they started Trazadone 50 mg at night. At this time diagnostics are repeated. The thyroid peroxidase antibody (TPO antibodies) are still elevated, therefore the doctors stated she would need a minimum of Vitamin D supplement at 50,000units/week.

Mom was given a break from the Cytoxan due to the shingles and in April 2011 she was due to go back to see Dr. Tornatore. Prior to that appointment I was researching HE to see if I could find any new information, something else that might help her. I found a random article that mentioned some success of treating HE with low dose Naltrexone (LDN) 4.5

mg/day. There was recent data showing an immunomodulatory effect.

Due to her symptoms of emotional lability currently the doctor decided to stop the Trazadone and start Prozac 10 mg/day. The first six weeks on LDN were amazing for her but unfortunately, she experienced an abrupt cessation of benefit from LDN after a brief viral illness. She was quite fatigued for a couple of weeks and took a short course of oral prednisone which helped her feel better.

By July 2011 she had very low energy, difficulty getting to sleep and staying asleep. She's very bothered by the tremor, it's almost always present now at rest. The tremor involves the voice, hands and legs. She was also complaining of frequent headaches involving the crown of her head. On exam she always has a positive Romberg with her eyes open, always hyperreflexia on bilateral lower extremities. The doctor moved to trying Primidone 50 mg for 3-4 days then will increase it to two times a day, if tolerated for the tremor. He also added Clonazepam.

In September, two months later, the new medication had stopped being effective for the tremor. Within the last two months she was beginning to get off balance easily and had experienced a couple of falls. She always falls to the right side. She also experienced rare episodes of disequilibrium that are almost a disembodied feeling with no premonitory state lasting less than or equivalent to 30 seconds and resolving spontaneously. She also complained of heat intolerance.

Since the Clonazepam was no longer working, the doctor then tried Topamax 50 mg twice daily for the tremor, frequent headaches, and episodic disequilibrium. By November 2011 my mom was complaining of additional numbness and tingling in her right hand with a lesser degree in the left hand. The tremor has been more intrusive, memory has not been good, more frequent headaches, and has lost twenty pounds in the last few months for no obvious reason. She says she doesn't feel hungry and forgets to eat, and she sleeps so much. At this point it is clear that her symptoms are returning, she has been off of Cytoxan for six months, they planned to restart it now that her symptoms were worsening.

In December they restarted the Cytoxan, by this time my mom was complaining of worsening tremors of hands, feet/legs, and voice. She kept a log of occurrences showing her doctor numerous occasions of numbness and tingling in both hands and feet, she was experiencing auras of the smell of burnt coffee, having few headaches – they decreased with the use of Topamax. The doctor decided to increase the Topamax dose to 100 mg twice daily for auras which he felt represented seizure activity.

In January 2012 she was able to report the tremor was much improved, only one or two brief auras since December. Her memory problems at this time are with retrieval type deficits. She has continued to lose weight – 35 pounds total now. Her doctor explained this by stating with HE – different parts of the brain are flared at different times. Right now the part of the brain that seemed to be inflamed was the part responsible for hunger and this area that would produce seizures if not managed properly.

One month later in February 2012 she was much improved – good control of vocal and extremity tremors, she was able to go to the gym for 90-120 minutes two to three times a week (by the way, important to note…she DOES NOT SWEAT even with a vigorous workout, this was also one of the initial symptoms retrospectively). She was experiencing no headaches or seizure activity. As the doctor increased the Cytoxan dose to her full dose of 1000mg, she experienced more side effects not enabling her to recover between treatments because the fatigue was overwhelming. They weaned back down on the dosage and side effects improved.

In November 2012 her symptoms were getting worse despite the Cytoxan every 4-6 weeks. The doctor added oral methotrexate 5 mg every third and fourth week following the Cytoxan infusion. This worked until February 2013. The frequent trips up the road are tough; physically, emotionally, and financially. The infusion itself is 6-8 hours long, she sleeps some of the day but come late afternoon she is chomping at the bit to just get out of there. In order to try something different the doctor thought she could stop the Cytoxan and start Leflunomide 10 mg/day. The problem came within one month – it caused thrombocytopenia and the medicine had to be discontinued. At this point the doctor decided to put the brakes on the Cytoxan and continue symptomatic therapy.

In July 2013 my mom's fatigue, balance, memory, tremors, olfactory auras, slow mental processing speed, word retrieval, have all been gradually worsening. Dr. Tornatore's team came up with a plan, by the way – she turned 65 years old in May 2013 and now that she is covered by Medicare it has opened doors to treatment options she didn't have with private insurance (that she paid for/worked for all of her life)! The plan is to do a plasma exchange transfusion (PLEX) for five cycles followed by Rituximab 375 mg/m2 one dose – to be repeated in six months. If they did not get good results, their plan B was to hit her with high dose Cytoxan for a three day infusion.

The end of July she arrived to Georgetown and was admitted, she had a double-lumen central line placed in her neck for the PLEX. The five day PLEX treatment consisted of three days on, a two day rest...followed by the last two days of exchange. This was followed the next day with the Rituximab infusion. For those who get Rituximab for the first time, just know that it has to be given very slowly and it is not unusual to experience some type of allergic response during the infusion. The doctors will slow down or sometimes stop the infusion treat with Benadryl and then continue on with the infusion as soon as your symptoms subside. My mom felt better within 48 hours; fatigue, gait, and tremor all much improved. She has been much more active since the PLEX/Rituximab treatment; she feels the best she has in over ten years! What wonderful results. Dr. Tornatore plans on repeating the Rituximab infusion in February 2014.

As I am sitting here writing this in November 2013 my mom is still feeling the benefits from the July treatment. Like everything else though, it's great at the beginning but starts to fade naturally as expected as time goes by. The more activity/stress she has the more exacerbated her symptoms are. I stumbled across the wonderful HE Facebook pages in July 2013 when mom was in the hospital and I have to say I undoubtedly learned so much more about HE from reading everyone's posts and comments than I EVER learned through medical references or physicians.

It's a wonderful thing to be able to tell my mom that she's not alone in this day to day fight in which her body attacks her brain; robbing her of the woman she was. For her to be able to identify with those that are experiencing the same symptoms helps validate her life as it is now. It lets her know she's not "crazy" with the way this horrible disease affects your emotions and personality making a person say, feel, and react in ways they never would have before HE attacked their brain.

The outsider may think she's in a bad mood or having a bad day, not understanding her disease. We didn't understand so many of these symptoms until connecting with other contributors of this wonderful book. My hope is that awareness sky rockets this disease and that physicians will pay attention and take the opportunity to learn about HE. I hope that more research is done to validate successful treatments so that insurance will cover them. I also want to acknowledge that for as devastating and debilitating this disease has been for my mom, through reading others stories we realize how fortunate she has been not to have experienced much worse episodic symptoms and times of medical crisis.

We are thankful to have been under the care of such a wonderful, smart (genius), genuinely caring physician in Dr. Carlo Tornatore and his Nurse Practitioner Erika Mitchell who never lets us down. We are also so thankful for our family and neighbors for their support. HE leaves a person feeling very isolated and alone, it takes a person's life away as they once knew it and presents frustrations in basic functioning. People have no idea. I hope after reading this book they have an appreciation for just how difficult every day is for an HE patient. My mom is a wonderful, caring, strong and independent woman and I am so proud of her for not giving up. My dad is an awesome support for her and I am so thankful he is the man he is, so caring, gentle and always supportive.

Laurie (age at diagnosis: 48)

I was 48 years old when I first developed noticeable HE symptoms. I am a published author and, at the time my symptoms first emerged, was an executive leading a global team at a large international consulting company. When I first began to realize something was wrong, I thought the symptoms were related to diabetes. (I was diagnosed with diabetes just a few months before I had my first HE "episode".)

My initial symptoms were primarily cognitive. At work, my role required me to develop a strategy for our team and lead the team. There was no instruction manual for the role.. I was the one who had to create the vision, the goals, and the road map of how we would get there. I had performed similar roles in the past (I had been at the company for 28 years) and the work had previously come fairly easy to me. I just had a knack for this type of work and for leading global teams. Over the 28 years I was with the company I had worked my way up from an assistant to an executive role. I was a top performer among my peer group, and was being groomed to move up to senior executive. I share all of that information not to brag but to provide context for the profoundness of the symptom "onset of cognitive issues".

It all started happening around June of 2011. I realized something was wrong when I began struggling to do a job that had been so easy for me in the past. It became difficult for me to put my thoughts together and almost impossible to create a strategy for my team. Also, suddenly it made me extremely nervous to give presentations to a global audience. I had never had a problem with this before.

When I would do presentations (luckily, during this timeframe I was giving the presentations over global conference calls), I had to write down everything that I was going to say and then read my notes when I was presenting. And, actually, I say that my symptoms appeared around in 2011, however, it was probably way earlier than this but this is when the symptoms became really profound to me. Cognitive issues probably began much earlier because as I reflect back now and talk with my husband, he has reminded me that even beginning at least a year before that, I told him that I had begun noticing that I wasn't thinking as quickly and as clearly as I had before and that I had to spend more time preparing for presentations than I had before.

I think the reason it became so profound to me in 2011 is because I had a new team and was dealing with new people at work and a new scope of work. For years previous to this, I had been managing a team under the same leadership for several years so the work was so familiar to me that I wasn't required to really stretch my thinking as I had done in the past. When I moved into the new role and had to really stretch my brain again, it's almost as if the brain I had before was no longer available to me.

The other symptoms that appeared at about this time were an onset of numbness in my right foot and leg, extreme fatigue, and an inability to exercise. I was riding my bike one day (following my son who was on a long run) and suddenly the muscles in my legs stopped working. I could go no further and felt I was going to collapse. I also felt like I couldn't breathe and started wheezing. After I made it home and rested, I recovered. So, I didn't go to the hospital. I followed up with my family doctor which led to the diagnosis of diabetes and I thought perhaps that was the reason for all of the problems.

My numbness continued to expand. My right arm and leg became very weak and numb. It became difficult at times to open a water bottle. I could no longer walk very far and I would sometimes drag my right leg.

I began having episodes of my neck feeling tight. It would come on suddenly, stay for awhile, and then go away. On January 24, 2012, my husband was driving me to my first neurologist appointment (to try to find out why I was having all of the numbness) when all of a sudden my neck got extremely tight (it felt as if I was about to lose the ability to breathe), and my face started going numb (starting with my chin and quickly moving up all the way up to my eye brows – it was almost like someone wiped my face with novacaine). My tongue went numb and the entire right side of my body went completely numb. This is the first time I had experienced anything like this. I thought I was having a stroke. So instead of going to my doctor, my husband drove me to the ER.

When I got to the ER, I couldn't speak and I couldn't stand/walk on my own. And, it seemed like I was in a different dimension. Everything felt weird. I knew where I was. I could hear people talking. I could see the fear on my husband's face. But, I couldn't really process it. It's almost like I was in a dream and I couldn't react to what was going on around me.

They took me for an MRI and found an arachnoid cyst on the left side of my brain. So, the doctors assumed this was causing my trouble (because the vast weakness was in my right leg and arm). I remained in the hospital for 4 days for monitoring to see if I would have another episode. I did not, however, I had residual issues and I would have minor episodes and my right arm remained weak. The neurosurgeon there wanted to operate. My husband and I wanted to get a second opinion.

When I was released from the hospital and went home, my family realized that my brain wasn't like it was before because I couldn't remember things that I knew before the "episode," such as where my son sat at the dinner table. And, when I would talk to people, I would give incorrect dates for well known information such as the year I graduated from high school. Also, I had difficulty with retaining information from conversations and struggled with procedural/instructional type of things such as following a recipe (I was an avid cook before my episode). Also, my right arm was so weak that I couldn't dice an onion on my own.

I searched for a second opinion on the "arachnoid cyst" diagnosis. Since I live in Houston, Texas and we have a world known medical center, I immediately started contacting neurosurgeons in the Medical Center. This is when I learned that most neurosurgeons won't see you without a referral. However, I was able to convince the nurse at a well-known neurosurgeon's office to let me see the surgeon. I think she felt sorry for me when I told her that I couldn't even dice an onion on my own.

When I met with the neurosurgeon, he listened to my story and immediately said that he thought there was something going on with my immune system. I was stunned because I had not even told him that I was diagnosed with Lupus SLE 30 years earlier. (I went into remission from SLE after steroid treatment 30 years ago and didn't think it was necessary to share that information with him since I was there to speak with him about my arachnoid cyst.) I knew right then that God put me with the right doctor. The doctor then referred me to see a Neurologist colleague of his. I met with the Neurologist and after running blood work, an EEG, MRI, and spinal tap, he diagnosed me with HE. I had the following abnormal blood work results:

- TPO
- Antiparietal Cell Antibody
- Microsomal Antibody

I was hospitalized in March 2012 for IV steroid treatment where I received 1 gram of IV steroids for 3 days, and I was released from hospital taking 60 mg of oral steroids. The weakness in my right arm and leg improved but didn't disappear. The doctors didn't really say what they thought about the results of the treatment. They just started the next round of treatments, which included Imuran. After several weeks of that I had to discontinue the treatment due to pancreas attack.

I then began Methotrexate with increasing dosage each week. After several weeks of treatment and on the same night I increased my dosage, I became violently ill with vomiting and diarrhea for 24 hours, I got large bruises on my feet, and was so weak, I could barely stand or walk to the bathroom, and I was short-of breath. I was hospitalized due to critically low potassium levels and dangerously inflamed pancreas.

As a result of treatment, I now have less frequent and less intense episodes but am still not back to my "normal" baseline. After the treatments were completed, my doctors felt I was going into remission even though I had these residual deficits.

The most significant symptom that remains with me today is cognitive issues that impair my ability to perform tasks. I struggle daily with the following:

- inability to retain details of conversations and written text
- difficulty following instructions and executing tasks
- inability to follow complex conversations
- remembering to take my medication
- inability to make decisions

Communication is sometimes difficult for me. At times, it is difficult for me to verbally explain my thoughts or provide detailed instructions and it's as if I can't find the right words to use. I don't like to talk on the phone anymore as I can't hear very well on the phone any more. I think my hearing has been affected. I plan to discuss this with my neurologist when I see him next. And, actually I don't talk much anymore. I mostly listen.

I also have short and long-term memory issues. I often incorrectly state key dates/facts (even things as "memorized" as my son's date of birth, my graduation date, etc.).

I lack the sense of urgency for anything. My intensity of my emotions have also changed. And, I have lost the desire for social activities or friends. I prefer to be in familiar place with my family.

I still experience the sudden onset of stoke/seizure-like symptoms and dizzy spells throughout the week (sometimes throughout the day). The intensity (and how long they last) varies by episode. The symptoms of the episodes can include some or all of the following:

- my neck gets tight (during more intense episodes, it gets so tight that it feels I will be unable to breath or swallow at any moment).
- my face goes numb - it feels like someone gave me a shot of Novacaine to my face
- my tongue and the roof of my mouth go numb
- dizziness (during more intense episodes it almost feels I'm in a different dimension)
- I feel as if I am moving in slow motion. My family says they can tell when I'm having one of these episodes because I look dazed and move slowly

- difficulty communicating verbally (I can talk but it is difficult to put thoughts together, communication is very choppy). This symptom occurs when the episode is one of the more intense ones.
- overall muscle weakness
- muscle twitches on the right side – this occurs sometimes as a warning to the episode but not always.

I also experience audio disturbances. On occasion, the fan in my bedroom sounds like a very loud engine. The disturbance usually lasts a minute or so but is disturbing when it happens.

I get sudden intense headaches that make it difficult to concentrate and perform tasks. I also have episodes of a sudden onset of confusion (and sometimes the inability to effectively communicate) in new, stressful, or very loud environments.

I have constant numbness in my right hand, right leg and foot, and muscle weakness on my right side.

I suffer from extreme fatigue, and feeling shaky – almost like the shaking is on the "inside". In fact, one night this was so intense that when I laid down, I felt like the bed was vibrating. That was a new symptom for me and it was very scary.

I have sleep disturbances – I usually fall asleep early because I am so tired, then I wake up around 2 or 3am, stay awake for a couple of hours and go back to bed around 5am and sleep until 8am.

I also have diabetes. Given all of the treatments I have had, I am just now getting my blood sugar numbers back under control.

All of these symptoms make it impossible to work. And, I can no longer drive. I can do some light housework and prepare simple meals. HE has drastically changed my life and who I was before. I was an executive who managed a large team, travelled internationally, my home office was our family "grand central station" with me managing everything and I loved it! I loved the fast pace of everything. I was very active. I loved water skiing, jogging, and I was an avid cook with dreams to open a restaurant when I retired. And because I loved to cook, my husband and I would entertain a lot.

Now, today, I just take life one day at a time. Because my muscles are so weak on my right side, I can no longer water ski and am no longer active. Because of my cognitive issues, I don't enjoy reading anymore because I can't retain what I have read. And, since I can no longer work, we are selling our dream house that we built 10 years ago (our lake house) to downsize and move to a more rural, simple lifestyle. While this is sad and I have gone through phases where I have felt a great sense of loss (and have cried a lot), I have faith that God is in control and there must be a reason for all of this.

God has given me a very supportive and loving husband and a wonderful family. Without them and without God, I could not have gone through this. And, while my life is very different today than it was before HE, I am grateful that I am still here with my family and that I have been here to watch my son grow up into the young man he has become.

I feel fortunate to have a neurologist who listens and considers my feelings and ideas. With him, I actually feel like I am part of the team trying to solve my health problem. From the beginning, he has worked together with my Rheumatologist and Endocrinologist to come up with a treatment plan.

I think with any major, chronic illness, there is a sense of loss. I've gone through the phases of "loss" – from denial to sadness and questioning why this has happened and, finally, acceptance. I still sometimes struggle with the emotions. I've broken down into tears many times over the past 2 years. But, I have come to accept that how I am today is likely my new "baseline". This is the new "me". So, I have been working on just trying to enjoy each day as much as I can.

I took my brain for granted before. More specifically, the fact that I could think and solve problems and retain details of conversations and stories. Now, I am more patient with people around me who maybe had difficulty remembering things or seem to move slowly. My pace in life has changed so my patience for others moving at a different pace has improved.

My prayer life has changed as well. When I read the Bible or some of the Christian books I had been reading before, I can't remember the details. And, sometimes I will start a prayer and not remember what I was praying and I get confused. So, I end up telling God I'm sorry but that I know He understands and accepts me for who I am. And, He knows what's on my heart.

I will continue to believe that God has a plan for me. So, HE hasn't changed my spiritual outlook, however, the illness (the cognitive issues) has changed the depth of my ability to worship and pray.

I'm optimistic because of my faith and because my husband (who is also my best friend who I have known since I was 14 years old) is by my side each step of the way.

One of the things that remains difficult for me is that it's extremely hard to explain some of the symptoms I've had. And, since everyone who has HE has different symptoms, it's sometimes easy to dismiss some of my symptoms. I did that while I was in a period of denial. Now, I realize that the only way I can get better and other people can get help is if we all keep track of our symptoms and share them so that we can learn from each other and doctors can learn.

I think the most difficult thing is that I expected to be well after treatments. I didn't expect to have residual deficits – the most difficult of which is that my brain has not returned to my normal baseline. And, it's strange to "know" the difference of who I am now and who I was before but not being able to do anything to fix it. That is where my faith and family come in. Jesus loves me just as I am and so does my family! That's what gets me through each day.

Another difficult thing I've had to face is the results of my neuropsychological tests. I've had two of these tests done as a result of HE. I hate them because during the test each time, it's like I experience a loss all over again. Because I go into the test optimistic and then as I am taking the test, it becomes very clear to me that my brain has changed… that I have lost some of my ability to process and remember. Each time when it hits me during the test, I cry. It's a very emotional experience. Unfortunately, both tests show that I am performing "below average". When I think about that today, I just think…. How is that possible? How can the brain just stop working the way it used to? HE is cruel that way. I look the same on the outside but have lost so much on the inside.

Now that I have moved into the acceptance phase of HE, I've been able to reflect on my family and how HE has affected them. They have lost something too. The wife my husband married changed. I'm not who I was. I can no longer engage him in political or theoretical debate. Now, I sit and listen and try to add what I can. But, he knows I won't remember the details of the discussion. I can no longer water ski or jetski with him. But, instead, I tag along and sit on the sidelines. He has accepted his "new" wife and his new life with compassion, love, and grace. A grace that only comes with true love. My son also has accepted the changes with love. He will be able to carry this experience with him through his life. Maybe the love that his father and I have for each other and how we have handled this experience will be a good example of marriage and that physical health does fade but true love endures.

James (age at diagnosis: 65)

As told by his daughter, "Weasie"

The story of my dad's illness begins in October 2008. He was born and raised in Appleton, Wisconsin, and that October he was in Madison, Wisconsin for a Badgers football game. He and my mother were at the hotel getting ready for the game when things started going downhill.

He was acting strangely, putting the sheets over the mirrors, walking up to the walls and touching them, as if he was pressing buttons, and he was not speaking normally. My mother felt she had no choice but to call an ambulance, which took him to Meriter Hospital.

While my dad was there they did an MRI to see if he was suffering from a stroke. He continued to do strange things like looking around the room as if he was following something, touching his pillow, talking nonsense. When the doctors looked at the MRI, they could not spot a stroke.

After many tests they did find that he had blockage in his carotid artery - about 96%. He just had a pin hole left open. He had the surgery for this, and there was a long waiting process.

After surgery, things seemed to be going okay. He had his appetite back, was sitting up in bed, and could almost carry on a full conversation. In the hospital, one day he was napping while the rest of my family went for a walk. I decided to stay with my dad so he would recognize someone when he woke up. I had a strange feeling about that day.

When he woke up, he looked around and when he looked at me it seemed like he was looking right through me. Something was definitely wrong.

The nurses continued coming in every hour and doing tests with him. He would follow their instructions, but he didn't always give them the answers they were looking for. It was like he would see something totally different than what they were showing him. Then he would start talking about being at St. Elizabeth's, which is a hospital in Appleton, where we lived. We would tell him we are in Madison and he would keep saying St. Elizabeth's.

Then he would talk to my mom saying things in conversations they had years ago. Throughout that day, things were recognizably wrong. At one point he told me to watch out because the spiders were going to get me. When I asked what spiders, he said "look, they are all over the ceiling, big blue fuzzy spiders."

The doctors wondered if he was suffering from alcohol withdrawal, but we knew that was not the case. They said he needed rest and as long as we were there he was not going to get it, so we left for the night.

The next day things got worse. He became combative, and was angry and punching and kicking, trying to take out his tubes. They had to strap my dad to his bed so he wouldn't hurt himself or anyone else. That was terrifying to see. He's my dad, not some animal.

This went on for days while they tried to diagnose him. They ran test after test, which irritated my dad even more because he kept being moved and pricked with needles. They told us that another MRI would be ideal, but with him being so combative they may not get an accurate reading because he would not be still enough.

Eventually they were able to get another MRI. They said they could see where he may have suffered a very minor stroke, but nothing that would cause this. They were at a loss so they ended up calling UW Madison Hospital, and he was transferred there.

After they got my dad settled in his new room at University Hospital, we were able to sit with him. They did not have him tied to his bed, and he was not acting combative but he was still acting very strange. At times he would look around the room as if following something, and then look right through you at other times.

Days passed again, and during this time there were a few really strange episodes. When they would have him sitting in a chair, he always wanted his pillow in his lap. He would hold the pillowcase at the seam with one hand and then act like he was hold a thread and needle in the other. He would make the motions as if he were sewing something. He would be in his own little world. We could not figure out why he would be doing that. My mom said he never sewed anything, not even a button on a shirt.

One day we were all in his room, and he was sitting in his chair, then out of nowhere he put his hand on his bed and started reciting something in a different language. In the middle of it, he ordered us all to join in. We all looked at each other and just started mumbling words. When he finished he went back to just sitting in his chair. The nurse in the room (he was under 24 hour observation from the nurses) told us he had just recited a prayer in fluent Latin - she studied the language in school. Again, we were all confused, how would he know Latin?

Then it clicked. My dad is a funeral director/mortician. His occupation consists of preparing a body to be shown, which requires the ability to sew. And he has also sat through multiples funerals through the years, and we are sure he has every prayer memorized in every language. In fact, my brother said they just recently had one that was done in Latin. But this was all still a little strange for us, he has never done this before. What was really amazing is that his speech was not the best since being in the hospital, so could not understand him most of the time.

More days went by, and there was still no diagnosis. Now, during this time he was having issues eating through a tube as well, so he had to undergo feeding tests. We would sit with him, show him pictures of family members and have him tell us who they were. He would slip on a few, but he knew most of them.

We were feeling afraid of Alzheimers, and in fact we heard one doctor mention that.

While my dad was in this hospital room, which was going on 2 weeks, after many, many tests, they still had nothing. They decided to move him to another room since they could not find anything seriously wrong with him. Shortly after being moved to his new room, my dad became combative again. This time, instead of locking him to his bed, they put these big white gloves on him, like boxing gloves so that he could not pull at anything, but he also couldn't itch his nose if it itched. This was so humiliating for him.

Days went by again and nothing changed. He just laid in bed, wouldn't talk, and slowly looked like he was given up on himself. He was scared. You could see it in his eyes, which scared the hell out of us. It was as if he knew what was wrong but couldn't tell us, or he was trying to tell us to give up.

They ran more tests. Nothing. Then, my dad was scheduled for a spinal tap. The evening before this, his student nurse that was sitting with him was thinking about my dad's case. This nurse had heard of Hashimoto's Encephalapothy and wondered if my dad should be tested. He knew it was a very rare disease, what could the odds be that this is what is wrong with my dad? Still, it seemed like it was worth testing for.

Guess what...my dad was finally diagnosed with something, something that is treatable, something that gave us hope. He had Hashimoto's Encephalopathy. Wow.

After the diagnosis, they still had to do tests, plus my dad was diabetic type II, so trying to find the right dosage of steroid meds for his HE was a little tricky. But finally, after many attempts, they found it.

My dad went through a long road of rehab in a hospital in Oshkosh, where we would visit him every day. But he was still not himself. Don't get me wrong - he could walk, talk, eat, etc. But all of it was like watching a child.

He did things out of the blue. One night he and I were sitting in the family room at the hospital and there was a chess board in front of us with the pieces on it. He picked one up and threw it in his mouth, then just sat there and looked at the wall.

They had to put the alarm on his belt because he was always trying to walk out the exit doors or get on the elevator. Ugh, he was there for days, but he got a little better each day. Finally we got the news of when we could bring him home: Christmas Eve.

On Christmas Eve, we each took turns to visit at my mom's house so we would not overwhelm him. He looked good, but still acted like a child at times. He needed help with pretty much everything. Each day was a struggle, for him and my mom, but it was for the good.

My mom got him a Wii system that he could play for motor skills. She got him headphones and movies so he could watch them without bothering her, as she worked from home as a medical transcriptionist. One of us kids would pick him up and go for a ride, or just sit and talk. He kept a journal for every day, and in it he wrote about what he did for the day, who visited, what he ate, etc...

The year before all of this started, my parents had been in Germany and fell in love with the Smart Car. My dad ordered one and it was being delivered in January. He was so excited, but it was sad because he couldn't drive it home. The day the Smart Car came to Milwaukee, my son was home from college so he rode along to pick the car up.

He took pictures of my dad sitting in the car, absolutely thrilled. My son drove the Smart Car back to Appleton with my dad as the passenger, and my son said all the way home my dad was honking the horn and waving at people. He thought he was the coolest thing out there.

We continued doing things as a family like we always have, and took him out on family field trips here and there. We all knew it was going to be a long road and he may possibly never be back to "normal," but he was alive and he is our dad.

Everything was going great, and we were all adapting to how things were and may always be. My mom and dad had a trip to New Orleans planned for March 2009, way before any of this started (in October 2008) and my dad was determined he was still going to make this trip. He wanted to go. My mom brought him to appointments with his doctors to make sure the doctors were okay with him taken this trip and to make sure she knew what to do in case of emergency. They gave him the go ahead and off they went with another couple, driving to New Orleans.

On their first night there, they decided to check out Bourbon Street. They visited the Funky Pirate and had a good time, and dad was amazed by all the strange surroundings. They went back to the hotel on St. Charles, and my mom was on the bed, with my dad standing by the vanity. He was struggling to get his coat off, which was a pullover. He had it up over his head, and then the worst imaginable thing happened: he lost his balance, which he had never fully recovered since he came down with HE. He fell backwards, and hit the back of his head on the hard floor. My mom can still hear that sound.

She screamed and yelled out for help. Their friends in the next room came over, and they managed to get my dad to the bed. The concierge, Tony, ran up to the room and he called 911. While they waited for the ambulance, Tony called his mother, who is a minister, and she came to say a prayer with all of them.

My dad was brought to Touro Hospital in New Orleans. We received the phone call back home, and my mom explained what happened. She said he seemed to be okay, but she wasn't sure. My brother flew out right away, and he called us with an update, saying that when he first got there Dad was speaking and able to walk with a cane. The next day my brother called and said it doesn't look good and we better come.

My sister, my son and I drove to New Orleans right away, straight through. We got there and my dad was hooked up to all types of machines, breathing tube in his mouth, everything. We had to take turns being with him, only 3 visitors at a time. The next day they talked with us, and said that he took a turn for the worse. His liver had failed and they said that if things keep shutting down, we will lose him.

The doctor made it sound like it was still possible he was going to pull through this. So we, as a family, had hope. That same night, my brother, my son and I drove back to Appleton, Wisconsin, straight through. My sister stayed with my mom.

My brother was now running the funeral home and had to tie up a few things. I also had to go to work and tie up a few things, and my son had to get back to college. I was able to get an FMLA leave with work, and in fact my boss insisted on it. My brother was ready to go back to New Orleans as well. We decided to meet at the funeral home at 4 am Sunday morning and leave from there.

New Orleans is a 15 hour drive. I had made this trip 2 times already. I drove first, about 4 hours, then my brother took over. We were about 3 more hours into the trip, leaving us with about 8 more hours of driving, when his phone rang.

It was my mom. My dad's heart had stopped and they were trying to start it. Then I heard her scream, loud. My dad passed away March 22nd, 2009 from a fall and hit to the back of his head. My brother and I drove, in silence, the 8 long hours to get to New Orleans.

We were ready as a family to fight this HE disease that was so rare, we were going to overcome it and have our dad back and with us every day. He was going to be at my son's college graduation, be there for the birth of his 1st great grandchild, for my daughter's high school graduation.

I know my dad did not die from HE, but I want him to be recognized for having had this rare disease. I want him part of the known cases, to maybe help others be diagnosed faster from symptoms like his, to be added to the number of people in the United States diagnosed with this disease that became part of our lives.

After he passed away, we were so focused on the fall, how he was treated at Touro Hospital. We didn't forget about his disease, but we no longer looked into it. He was gone.

I want to make up for that and acknowledge it, and hopefully help the study of this disease with his story. If there was one thing that my dad was, it was a hard worker.

He worked very hard at being the man he was. He was a unique man as well, I don't want people to only know him as dying from a fall, I want people to know his short journey with this rare disease. He was a hero in my eyes.

Allison

My journey with HE started on September 11th, 2009, when I was carted out of work on a gurney. Within 30 minutes, I had lost my vision, ability to speak, had numbness on the whole right side of my body and was basically freaking out.

I was only 26 years old. I had no idea what was happening to me, but the scariest thing was that no one else could figure out what was wrong either.

I had to take disability from work, and I spent days curled up on the floor, unable to walk or properly articulate and only having vision from one eye. After a couple weeks of failed migraine medications, my doctor (neurologist) tried a prednisone pack. I got my vision back! Finally progress!

He did some research, checked my anti-thyroid antibodies and diagnosed me with Hashimoto's Encephalopathy. I followed the typical treatment plan… high dose IV methylprednisolone in the hospital, 1g a day for 5 days. I had significantly improved. But I was still suffering from a host of symptoms, in addition to the new side effects from continuing high dose oral prednisone.

I tried IVIG, Plasmapheresis and so many other drugs and treatments to no acceptable satisfaction of life. At one point, I was on somewhere around 21 different medications.

I began researching almost non-stop. I started a website at www.henotebook.wordpress.com to collect my thoughts, knowing my memory had become so bad, and also hoping my efforts may help other people suffering like I was.

I decided high dose steroids were not the final answer. Steroids are a double edged sword. Yes, they suppressed my immune system, but my heart rate was out of control, my skin, eyes and adrenal gland was suffering. And at one point,

I DIDN'T SLEEP AT ALL FOR 3 MONTHS! Literally... not a wink.

I tapered down fairly quickly. I went into withdrawal, so I was feeling a different kind of sick all the time, but I finally made it down to no prednisone... And then I went into adrenal crisis. Yup, the high dose steroids over the years had basically killed my adrenal gland, so I wasn't producing cortisol to live. So one of my side effects was needing to take a small amount of steroids every day since my body no longer produced it.

For the seizures and steroid induced anxiety, I used clonazepam. When I first started it, I remember saying, "It just makes me feel normal." I've been up (way up) on the dose and down. But nothing else works for my seizures. I tried 6 different antiepileptic medications (oxcarbazepine, valproic acid, depakote, and some others I can't remember). All had horrific side effects. I felt locked inside myself, unable to access most of my brain, unable to communicate effectively, and I lost the desire to live. My husband left me at this time. He couldn't deal with me being so sick. I don't know what it's like to watch your spouse degrade into a vegetable. So it's not my job to judge, but for those of you going through this and those watching a loved one go through this, try to focus on the love and the hope for health, rather than the illness.

Moving on, once my doctor saw what the antiepileptics were doing to me and how I couldn't take it anymore, he put me back on clonazepam. THANK GOD!

I had come across Imuran (azathioprine) in my research. There wasn't much about it regarding treating symptoms like mine, but I figured it was worth a try. It was hard convincing my doctor to put me on a chemo for liver transplant patients, but it was the best thing I did for my health. I started at the max dose for my weight (dosage is based on weight) and tapered down. I relapsed at 50mg, so went back up to 100mg.

The combination of 20mg hydrocortisone (=4mg prednisone), 4mg clonazepam and 100mg azathioprine had me finally feeling healthy!

I went back at work as an electrical engineer. I resumed caving, rock climbing, running, and hiking. I still have a touch of speech and memory difficulty, but I have learned ways to help, like keeping a notebook to remember stuff and asking people to NOT finish my sentences and just let me take a second to get the words out (for those lost speech moments at work, I just pretend I am thinking of something brilliant to say, lol). The only thing that is a significant problem is the headaches are still quite terrible. Oh well, I'll take that over fetal position on the bathroom floor!

I had been wanting to have a child, and made the decision to try after I happened to find research on women taking azathioprine (the one drug the docs worried about, and the one I was too scared to stop taking). Aside from a high increase in pre-term birth, the statistics for azathioprine babies were quite close to average statistics for birth defects (my biggest concern).

It was hard just to make the decision to actually risk a pregnancy, but actually getting pregnant proved to be difficult as well.

I tried the old fashioned way for 6 months but it was unsuccessful.

Prior to starting Imuran, I had had no idea what it would do to my body, so I decided to begin the in vitro fertilization process by harvesting my mature eggs. Many people and a few doctors told me this was a bad idea to go through the hormone injections and the toll it takes on my body, but I wanted to have eggs just in case I needed them for the future, so I went ahead and did it.

It sure wasn't an easy process. But it wasn't because of the HE. I produced 3 times the amount of eggs an average woman does in this process. I went into hyper ovarian stimulation syndrome, and my ovaries swelled to the size of grapefruits. Terribly painful. Harvesting was the biggest nightmare (I'll spare the details), but I've got 35 good eggs in the freezer just in case I need them. :)

I saw several doctors about pregnancy. The docs were split 50/50 if it was safe to do it (for me and the baby). They were both concerned about the drugs I was taking (mostly the azathioprine) as well as some evidence that autoimmune diseases usually flare up during pregnancy. My sister's Chrohn's flares up badly when she is pregnant, so I was disappointed thinking

I could never safely get pregnant, but I still wanted desperately to be a mother. I tried adoption and surrogacy and ended up heartbroken each time it didn't work out.

By October 2012 I had been attempting pregnancy for 8 months. I'd been taking the fertility medications, ovulating 3+ eggs per month. In September I felt a lot of cramping at the time an egg should've implanted. I had an ultrasound and blood test to check hormone levels, and we were fairly sure I had conceived. Unfortunately, I developed a sinus infection, and my job switched my shifts, all causing a lot of stress. I got terrible headaches, very bad cramping, followed by a heavy period. Very possibly I had a very early term miscarriage. After that, I decided to do in vitro fertilization, to increase my chances of getting pregnant to a drastic 60%.

In order to avoid an emotional and costly miscarriage after IVF, I needed to destress. I changed jobs (within the same company) and put school on hold. I was doing too much for a "normal" person, let alone a person with HE… and one trying to get pregnant.

Flash forward to March 2013. I knew I wasn't supposed to announce anything until 14-16 weeks, but I announced on my HE website that I was pregnant, about 6 weeks! Seeing the baby's heartbeat on the ultrasound was the happiest moment of my life. I knew it was a VERY high risk pregnancy and I had already been put on bedrest twice and had to go to the hospital.

I received weekly ultrasounds and blood tests, and had to give myself daily hormone injections because my adrenal gland and thyroid weren't working properly to support my uterine lining. I couldn't continue to work at my job (due to the strain on my abdomen).

I was fearful every moment of losing the baby, which is why I was hesitant to tell anyone. But I had shared my ups and downs with HE on the website, so I thought I might as well share my ups and downs as a pregnant woman with HE.

By the time I entered my second trimester I was still having pregnancy emergencies like severe pain and bleeding. Nevertheless, the baby continued growing and developing normally, and was VERY active. I'd heard so many people say how beautiful and delightful pregnancy is... Well it sure hadn't been for me. I hadn't been able to work, I was frequently on bed rest, and the "pregnancy symptoms" seemed to be magnified in me. Although I was ecstatic to have a child, pregnancy had been awful. And I still had so long to go! Although I had been told by others with HE that pregnancy was difficult any typically ended in miscarriage I had taken the chance because I had exhausted my other options (like adoption and surrogacy). I didn't regret my decision to get pregnant, but I still certainly didn't expect it to be so difficult and painful.

As I approached my third trimester I was taking 20mg hydrocortisone, 4mg clonazepam, and 100mg azathioprine daily, plus the prenatals and the occasional vicodin for severe headaches. The specialist decided these medications at these levels were not of a big enough risk to my baby to be concerned. I had an anatomy scan ultrasound, and my baby was shown to be very healthy. His organs were the right size and functioning normally, his bones were well formed, his skin and neck were the right size. He was VERY active and kicked all the time! He was also much BIGGER than average.

The doctor said "He's long, tall and thin, just like his Mom." He was also estimated to be almost half a pound heavier than most babies at this stage. What's interesting is that azathioprine use during pregnancy results in low birth weight 50% of the time. I eat an all organic, gluten-free diet with lots of fruits and vegetables, and drink lots of water. I do believe all that was helping. I was gaining the recommended weight for pregnancy and had not failed any of the blood pressure tests or sugar tests.

On October 29, 2013, my son, James, was born at 7:23pm EST. He weighed 8 pounds 3 ounces, and was 20 inches long. It had been an incredibly emotional and scary ride, but it was over and I have a very healthy, big, strong boy. I could write a book about the birth and my emotions, but I'll keep it short and pointed. The birth was induced at 39 weeks. The baby was fully developed and large (via the ultrasounds) and I had been having terrible pain, specifically the common nerve pain associated with a baby that has dropped for birth. So the decision to induce was for my health and to prevent any possible HE complications.

My water was broken and I was given a low starting dose of pitocin. I immediately went into very strong labor. They halved the dose of pitocin and gave me demerol to help me get through the contractions. About 5 hours later, I gave birth and held a screaming baby boy. I didn't need a doctor to tell me his lungs were fine, but that had been a concern due to the HE drugs. His lungs and birth weight were better than average, despite the 100mg azathioprine, 20mg hydrocortisone and 4mg clonazepam daily. He passed all his tests and measurements perfectly. Despite the medications, I had eaten well, taken prenatal vitamins and exercised. A healthy lifestyle helped to beat the high odds of complications.

The hospital recommended I not breastfeed due to the clonazepam, but I had gone to a specialist and also looked up the risks myself and I decided to breastfeed. He has been breastfeeding for a bit over 2 weeks now and he is gaining weight normally and has no respiratory issues. I do supplement with formula when I cannot breastfeed to give him the proper amount for feedings. So baby is wonderful and healthy. I did have one complication of hemorrhaging very badly one week after birth. There was a bit of placenta left over after birth and I had to have a D&C to remove it. I lost A LOT of blood so I was admitted to the hospital overnight, and it after just over a week I was still working on the postpartum anemia.

My new doctor now wants to wean me off the hydrocortisone AND clonazepam, which is terrifying since my cocktail has worked so well for so long, but that is the new struggle now that I'm back to being a single person in this body. I'm thrilled I'm finally a mother, and I'm beyond relieved my baby boy is happy and healthy.

Larry (age at diagnosis: 56)

I am by profession a writer, editor, teacher, speaker, and organizational executive.

November 2011-April 2012

The first time I noticed something strange going on was in November 2011, when I began to think that I was reading special meaning into student papers I was grading, thinking that I had read hidden comments about me.

Soon after that, I started to think that people on television were actually speaking to me by making all kinds of odd references that seemed to have relevance to things I had recently done or said or was currently doing while watching television.

In December 2011, I was reminded of the story of *The Little Prince* and began to think that it had some immediate relevance for me.

Also in January 2012, I had my first major episode of what would later be diagnosed as Hashimoto's Encephalopathy, in which I experienced in a fearful way a paranoid delusion that someone was trying to kill me. I was sick with laryngitis and bronchitis and went to the emergency room. There, I believed that the medical personnel were possibly trying to kill me, or that someone pretending to be a medical caregiver wanted to do so.

The first clue as to what was going on, and which eventually put us on the right track to figuring out a correct diagnosis, was that I was given a prescription for Prednisone to treat the laryngitis and bronchitis. Within several days my laryngitis and bronchitis began to improve. The big surprise was that it seemed as if my head suddenly cleared as well. All of the thoughts of someone out to get me, of people on TV talking specifically to me, and related thoughts suddenly seemed to evaporate. Still, it would be another four months before we had an accurate diagnosis, and a great many symptoms and uncertainties occurred during that time.

On May 2, 2012, I wrote the following letter to the six different doctors whom I had seen from December 2011 to May 2012, as I went from one doctor to another in an effort to figure out what was going on. The following letter offers a good account of the symptoms I experienced during that period, the doctors I saw, and related matters.

May 2, 2012

Dear Drs. W (Rheumatologist), V (Neurologist), P (Psychiatrist), B (Endocrinologist), M (General Practitioner), and L (Psychologist):

I am writing, in part, to thank each of you for your medical support. Each of you has played a part in uncovering pieces of the puzzle that has now led to a diagnosis. I am most grateful.

I am also writing in an effort to share this recent diagnosis with all of you, especially as it pertains to my past and future visits with each of you. I am going into considerable detail here and will be grateful if each of you will take the time to read this letter.

Following my visit with Dr. W on April 25, on April 27, 2012 I received a call from Dr. W's office with a diagnosis of Hashimoto's Encephalopathy (HE), which I have since learned is a very rare illness. As I have begun to read about it, it also seems to make sense of a great many symptoms that I have had off-and-on for months, or even longer.

On April 26, 2012, I also saw Dr. V. She reviewed the test results that she had ordered and mentioned two test results in particular: a Thyroid Peroxidase AB value of 118 and a Thyroglobulin Panel value of 103. Based upon that, plus other symptoms, I think Dr. V mentioned the possibility of my having: Steroid-Responsive Encephalopathy Associated with Autoimmune Thyroiditis (SREAT), which I now understand to be another name for Hashimoto's Encephalopathy.

Among the lists of symptoms for HE/SREAT, I see numerous symptoms that I have experienced off-and-on, over time. Here are the ones that I have been dealing with—

1. Short Term Memory Loss—intermittent (Long term memory and cognition appear unaffected)

2. Difficulty Concentrating–frequent

3. Fatigue–constant

4. Perceived smells that aren't present in my environment–occasional

5. Involuntary movements (especially with my neck)–occasional

6. Personality Change (suspicious, fearful, anxious)—in recent months

7. Muscle weakness (especially with my arms and hands)—occasionally. For some reason, toweling off after a shower has felt especially difficult to do at times. Towel feels strangely heavy and awkward in my hands and arms.

8. Difficulty staying awake–occasionally

9. Difficulty standing up–occasionally

10. Difficulty walking–rarely

11. Confusion–occasionally

12. Stuttering—two specific instances where I stuttered and could not speak intelligibly for 30-60 minutes. Remained conscious and aware throughout.

13. Bizarre Dreams (in one instance, talking and singing gibberish out loud for 30 minutes one night, I am told. Seemed like someone or something was standing behind me, touching my head, teaching me their language. Son audiotaped 2 minutes of it)–occasionally

14. Constant high-pitched noise in my left ear (two months and counting). Really annoying.

15. Occasional pressure or pain in my left ear.

16. Psychosis/Ideas of Reference (frequently thinking that things I had read or saw on television were somehow said for my benefit, as if someone was either watching me or trying to give me clues to some mystery that I was supposed to solve. Began in November 2011. Has stopped.
17. Frequent instances while driving of having my eyes rapidly scanning auto license plates as they drive past me, also reading words, letters, numbers on the sides of trucks. Sometimes consciously doing so, other times I became aware that I had been doing it for a while.
18. Tremors–Occasionally
19. Uncertain, but seems like I have been losing hair on my lower legs.—Six months?
20. Intentional tremors (instances of this when picking up cups of coffee)–Occasionally
21. Generally speaking, I have always felt too warm. At night, I would sleep without a sheet or cover. In recent weeks, I have felt cold, shivering and have been sleeping under a comforter. Last two nights that seemed to switch back and I have felt too warm. Wondering if this is thyroid-related, and should I be taking Levoxyl?
22. Speech difficulties–Occasionally
23. Difficulty retaining information (especially people's names)–Frequently
24. Seriously delusional/paranoid for two or three days in March and wound up at Stress Center for four days. While I

was conscious that I was thinking of bizarre possibilities (what-if's?), it seemed that I couldn't discount them enough as being only remote possibilities, and so they seemed like they were either happening, or on the verge of happening. Mostly, I knew they couldn't be real, but they felt all too real as possibilities. Among the things that I imagined during that time: That alien creatures were hiding and about to take over the world; that this was known by our government and plans were underway to take some people to hidden underground bunkers where we would have to live for years; I imagined that someone was trying to kill me; I imagined that someone was about to give me millions of dollars; I imagined that my wife was having an affair; I imagined that someone was trying to give me clues to help me solve these and other mysteries; I imagined that someone was watching and listening to us through our TV's and computers; I imagined that I was being tested for some secret or cosmic reason; I had unusual instances of smelling things that were not present (I believed that our house, and then my car, and then everywhere outside had an unpleasant musty odor for about 48 hours)—part of the delusion that alien creatures were transforming our environment into one where they could live and breathe, but we couldn't. For months, I have also smelled frequently some strong, flowery perfume smell that I recall my Grandmother wearing when I was a kid. Other strange smells that were not there, especially the burning smell of smoke, or of something electrical burning.

25. On the second day at the Stress Center, I was put on Geodon (40 MG x2, in am and pm). I think I was also taking an anti-inflammatory of some kind. Within one-day, it seemed as if nearly all of these imaginings and ideas of references stopped. Unfortunately, it also made it extraordinarily hard to stay awake. I felt like I was often on the verge of falling asleep. I also had breathing problems with it the first night that I took it. The breathing problems stopped after one night, but I continued to feel like I was constantly on the verge of falling asleep, including while driving.

26. April 10-19, I drove to Wisconsin and Minnesota where I gave a series of five presentations as part of my work (two 90-minute talks; two two-hour talks; and a 7-hour workshop.) Despite feeling as if I wanted to sleep, I made it through all of them, plus some meetings.

27. On April 27, in consultation with Dr. P, I dropped down to taking one Geodon at night. That has helped so that I no longer feel like I am on the verge of falling asleep during the day. In the past week, I have had only a few brief instances of wondering whether there was some deeper meaning in something that I was reading.

28. Still feeling waves of emotion wash over me (last six months).

29. It is interesting that both the Prednisone in January, and the Geodon in April, seemed to stop these ideas of reference/delusions. What does it mean that an anti-inflammatory and an anti-psychotic would have the same effect?

There are also other symptoms or events that have occurred over time, and which I want to list here in case any of this has any meaning to you.—

- Nail bed underneath my right big toe turned blue in early April 2012, and it remains blue as of May 2, 2012. Days before I noticed it had turned blue, I felt occasional "electric shocks" at the end of that toe. I did not stub it or drop anything on it.
- I am reminded that I have occasionally felt similar electric shocks in my feet, legs, thighs, arms, and fingers, strong enough to make me jump, or let out a yell. Not static electricity either—feels like it is coming from underneath my skin.
- Over the past year, my eyesight is as if I am looking through a watery film. I see many things floating across my line of sight. Mostly four different shapes: Hair like, tangled shape, spiderlike (definitely moving legs), and tiny indigo-colored dots.
- Treated for Laryngitis and Bronchitis in January 2012. Took Prednisone and an antibiotic for this and felt much better in all ways for 4-6 weeks. No "Ideas of Reference" during that time, which I had been having constantly previous two months (late-November to mid-January). By early March, these ideas of reference and delusions returned, stronger than before. I also began smelling things that were not there, and I was

aware of my eyes darting to look at license plates and other words/numbers on trucks and cars.

- Diagnosed with Type 2 Diabetes in Summer 2011. Treated with low-carbohydrate diet and diabetes numbers dropped back into normal range in year-end testing.
- Treated for Colitis in May 2011. No bacterial cause could be identified. While taking antibiotic medication for this I drove to Dallas, Texas. After driving long day, I got out of car and into hotel. Looked in bathroom mirror and saw a strange bright red rash on my face. As I recall, it went away after 1 or 2 days. I might also have been taking an anti-inflammatory at the time (not sure). Remember wondering whether combination of sun and meds could have caused the rash. It was a very bright red color, like little dots.
- One of the tests run in May 2011 (an ANA test, I think) showed elevated levels of inflammation. This eventually led to my seeing Dr. W; and, along with his own diagnosis, led Dr. P to think that I had something that was not a psychiatric-caused problem. I believe the elevated ANA result is also what caused Dr. M to prescribe the Meloxicam that I have been taking since sometime in 2011.
- In recent years, I have frequently experienced frequent tearing out of my outside right eye. Eyes are also

frequently burning so much that I have to wipe with tissue before they tear up completely. Occasional problem when it happens while driving.

- Diagnosed with Sleep Apnea around 2004. (Tried CPAP, BiPAP, and dental device but couldn't tolerate any of them. Eventually began sleeping on foam wedge pillow and taking Provigil and have felt rested enough to function okay for last half-dozen years. Dr. H.
- Treated for what I was told was Vasculitis at some point in early 2000's. Dr. R.
- Knee-surgery for torn meniscus around 2005.
- Diagnosed with various allergies around 2001 (Dust mites, Cat dander, various grasses, molds, trees). Dr. W (I think).
- Treated for Pleurisy in 2000. Dr. R.
- Treated numerous times for inflammation of various parts of my body with no apparent cause: swollen back, feet, ankles, knuckles. Mostly at Immediate Care Centers (going back many years).
- Treated with something called Sporanox for what I was told was some rare South American fungus that ate a hole in my right arm back around 1995. Took months to heal over. The fungus was associated with South American rose-handlers, as I recall. I had never been to South America, nor did we have any rose bushes. Dr. G (skin specialist).

- Epstein-Barr Virus in 1974. Dr. A.
- For what it's worth, I do not believe I have ever had a headache in my life.
- Mother had TB in 1954. I was born in 1955. Could anything in her treatment have affected my genetic development in some way?
- Father had Polio, Diabetes, Congestive Heart Failure.
- Mother had Rheumatoid Arthritis, Kidney Disease, Congestive Heart Failure, and COPD.
- As of May 2, 2012, I am taking these medications at the present time—
- Losartin-HCTZ 50-12.5 MG Tab (x1/day), Cholestorol-lowering–M
- Meloxicam 15 MG Tab (x1/day)—Anti-inflammatory, M
- Pravastatin Sodium 40 MG Tab (x1/day), Blood pressure–M
- Provigil/Modafinil 200 MG Tab (x1/day)—Wakefulness, M
- Advair 100/50 (1 puff x2/day)—Asthma, M
- Prednisone 10 MG (x3/10 days; x2/10 days; x1/10 days), HE–W
- Geodon/Ziprasidone HCL 40 MG Cap (x1/night)—Psychiatric (weaning) P

In addition to seeing all five of you, in recent months I have had scattered visits to four different E.R.'s 1(stuttering/gibberish,

MRI), 2 (MRI), 3 (diagnosed with Colitis, couldn't find a cause; showed elevated ANA results), and 4 (in Madison, Wisconsin where, sick with bronchitis and laryngitis/difficulty breathing/anxious, ran numerous tests, not sure what at this time, other than they gave me two nebulizer treatments, a bag of saline, and told me some test that they did while I was there showed benign "nodules" in my upper chest and to tell my doctor about them). Several visits to the Immediate Care Center, including one in January just a few days after being at the Madison ER. It was at the Immediate Care Center where I was given a prescription of Prednisone and immediately noticed that all the bizarre thoughts disappeared within a day or two of starting to take the Prednisone pills.

April 2012-March 2013

My ongoing treatment for the next year (April 2012 to March 2013) found me seeing both my Endocrinologist (Dr. B) and my Neurologist (Dr. V). Dr. V had been the person to first identify this as Hashimoto's Encephalopathy, based upon various blood tests, MRI's, and other tests that had been done. This illness seems to straddle neurology and endocrinology, and she had referred me to Dr. B for further testing and treatment.

During this twelve month period I saw Dr. B three or four times and Dr. V twice, I believe. Dr. B had me on tapering doses of Prednisone on several different occasions. However, within a few weeks of stopping the Prednisone my symptoms had returned and so she resumed the use of it. At various times I was on as much as 30 mg. of Prednisone, though generally speaking it was either 20 mg. or 10 mg. for much of that time, before going off of it for a short time. It became clear that Prednisone seems to keep it mostly in check, but that it returns if I am not taking Prednisone.

However, nothing had prepared me for my first real "flare-up" of HE, which returned with a vengeance in March 2013.

In mid-March of 2013, I once again began to experience both the physical and psychiatric manifestations of Hashimoto's Encephalopathy. Despite the experience of having gone through this the first time around, it didn't seem to help much and I found myself within a few days back in the hospital, though this time simply admitted to the hospital, for eight days of testing and treatments.

During this stay, I experienced a great many delusions and hallucinations—far too many to even list at this moment. Most were truly frightening, though some were exciting, even funny at times.

While I was not too lucid during the early days of my hospital stay in mid-March, 2013 it was decided that I would undergo an IV treatment of Prednisone, and I received 1 gram of Prednisone a day for three days. When that didn't seem to make a difference, I was then given a five-treatment course of plasmapheresis. This did seem to make a difference for me, and while I was still a bit shaky from the whole experience, I was discharged on March 26, 2013 and returned home, where I continued to heal, and where I am feeling pretty much back to normal as of this writing (April 26, 2013).

While in the hospital, I was prescribed an anti-psychotic medication called Abilify, which I am continuing to take. It seems clear from the studies that my doctors and I have been reading that Hashimoto's Encephalopathy seems to come either with physical-symptoms only or physical-and-psychiatric symptoms, and I seem to fall into the second category.

At the moment (for the past month), my symptoms have gone away. I continue to work, to drive, and to lead a normal life. I am married and my wife and I have two adult children who no longer live at home.

As of this writing, I am taking 40 mg. of Prednisone a day.

Earlier in this piece, I mentioned that at the time of my initial HE experience, the nail bed underneath my big toe on my right foot had hurt, then turned blue, then black, then the nail eventually fell off, to be replaced by a new toenail. I hadn't stubbed my toe and I didn't drop anything on it. I mentioned this to my doctors and wondered if it might also be a symptom of my HE, but that suggestion was dismissed as unlikely and no one knew what might have caused it.

For the record, and in case anyone reading this has had a similar experience, several weeks ago this happened to me for a second time. It did so in conjunction with my major flare-up of HE. While I did not have the electrical shock feeling that I had first time around, this time I felt discomfort in my big toe, and it was easy to see that my toe was swollen. The cuticle of the toe became red, and the nail underneath turned red, and has now turned blue and is getting darker. If it follows the path of the first time, I expect that it will continue to turn black and that eventually my toenail will fall off, to be replaced by another one. I am 100% certain that I did not stub my toe or drop anything on it. In addition, with this second occurrence in conjunction with Hashimoto's, I am pretty well-convinced that I have identified a symptom that, at least for me, is somehow connected to my own HE. Would like to know if anyone else has or has had a similar experience!

Also, at the moment, the primary way that HE impacts my daily life is that as a result of having the IV treatments in March 2013, it induced in me Type 2 Diabetes so that I am presently having to test my blood glucose four times a day, and to give myself insulin injections—generally once or twice a day. I am working closely with my Endocrinologist and we are hopeful that this is just a temporary problem and that through a low carb/low calorie diet, plus exercise, plus weight loss, plus using insulin as needed, I will eventually reach a point where insulin will no longer be needed as a treatment. I hope so.

My reaction to HE is one of amazement. I am amazed that such an illness exists; that so few people have it; and, that I am one of those who does have it. I find myself wanting to learn more about it, and wanting to encourage medical researchers and professionals to search for a cause and a cure if one can be found.

My outlook on life remains very positive. My experiences have made me feel greater empathy for anyone who suffers from any kind of illness, and particularly those who have HE.

I would like to add that In December 2012, in advance of scheduled appointments with my Endocrinologist and Neurologist, I wrote a second letter bringing them up-to-date on matters that had occurred in 2012. What follows is that letter—

To: Dr. B, Endocrinology
Dr. V, Neurology

From: L

Date: Dec. 26, 2012

In anticipation of my upcoming appointments with each of you [9:45 a.m., Dec. 27, 2012, Dr. V; 8:40 a.m., Feb. 4, 2013, Dr.] I wanted to provide you with this update…

…From early November to early December, the only HE/SREAT symptoms that I continued to experience involved my involuntarily saying words (usually "yes," "no," or "what;" or making sounds (usually a "Sssss" sound). This nearly always occurring at night between the time I put my head on the pillow and the time I would fall sleep. Most other symptoms that I experienced earlier in the year [detailed in my letter to you of May 2, 2012] disappeared.

Within a period of several days, around December 8, 2012, the following symptoms returned: feelings of suspicion, high pitched hum in my left ear, involuntary jerking of my body when lying down, difficulty concentrating, perceiving smells not in my environment (usually either a burning electrical odor, or sometimes a kind of sweet perfume fragrance from forty years ago that I recall my Grandmother wore), disturbed sleep, trouble with my hands (repeated feeling of my hands cramping up, but only when holding/using a washcloth!). I had leftover Prednisone from my previous prescription and, based upon what I have been reading about HE/SREAT, I resumed taking it on December 10—taking 10 mg. in the morning and 10 mg. at night (20 mg. total). Within a few days, nearly all of the symptoms had disappeared. The one symptom that remains now is the high-pitched sound in my left ear, which I believe began in March.

As I write this on December 26, 2012, I feel great. All symptoms save one (the high-pitched sound in my left ear) have disappeared. I have been taking 20 mg. of Prednisone for two weeks. On Jan. 3, I will head up to Minnesota where I will be teaching a month-long course, returning home on Feb. 2. Then, on Feb. 5, I fly to California for a week of meetings and speaking before returning home on Feb. 11. I want to continue to feel good and to be able to function well during this period. I imagine that the best way to insure that is for me to continue to take 20 mg. of Prednisone a day—at least until I return on Feb. 11.

I felt traumatized earlier this year by my HE/SREAT experiences with psychosis/paranoia, delusional thinking, and the many other physical symptoms that I had earlier this year and which led to my spending five days in the Stress Center in March 2012. I do not ever want to repeat that experience—neither that array of symptoms, nor being hospitalized like that…"

In terms of other illnesses in my medical history, over the years I have had:

- Colitis
- Arthritis
- Asthma
- Allergies
- Vasculitis
- Sensitivities to smoke, some cleaning products
- Bronchitis
- Diabetes
- Dry eyes
- High blood pressure
- Joint pain
- Obesity
- Sinusitis
- Pleurisy
- Numerous instances of inflammation of back, ankles, feet

In addition, in the 1990s, I was treated for what I was told was an uncommon fungal infection on my arm by Dr.

G. He did some kind of culture test and determined that it was a rare infection mostly found among South American rose growers. I know that it was treated with something called Sporanox (Itraconazole) and that it eventually healed. The infection may have been called something like Sporatrichosis.

In 1970s, Dr. A treated me for Epstein-Barr.

November 2013

It is now November 10, 2013. In the intervening seven months since I first wrote this piece, my health has improved. I was weaned off Prednisone and, within a few months, my blood sugar dropped back into normal range so that I no longer have to give myself insulin shots. As a result of my hospital experience in March 2013, I can only urge caution when taking massive doses of prednisone. I tend to believe that it was the series of plasmapheresis treatments that finally resolved my flare-up back in May, but I don't think anyone knows for sure. The prednisone has since been replaced by a drug called Imuran (Azithiopine), used in the treatment of autoimmune diseases. Three months in, and this seems to be working, and without the side effects that go with taking Prednisone. I have not experienced any return of physical or psychiatric symptoms.

I feel lucky that I continue to be able to work (teach, write, edit, speak, travel, drive). There were times in the past two years where I feared that I might not be able to do any of it.

I am cautiously optimistic and hopeful that the Imuran will continue to keep my HE in-check. My doctor's advice that I should plan on taking Imuran for the next five years before any consideration of weaning me off of it.

For those diagnosed with HE/SREAT, I hope that you have found (or will find) a good Endocrinologist and/or Neurologist—someone who is open to doing the research and ordering the tests needed to accurately diagnose this syndrome. I wish you the best.

Christine

My initial symptoms were those associated with hypothyroidism: I felt cold, was tired, and seemed to be slow in my thinking. Eventually I had to quit my job because I couldn't keep up. Then I began to have dizzy spells. I became concerned. All this was slowly building. One day I collapsed in the shower. But, the strange thing was, I really didn't faint. I just collapsed, retaining consciousness.

I was having a problem with dizziness so I went to the doctor. While I was there I had a spell and was transported to the hospital. I was bedridden after that. I had "non-epileptic" seizures if there was a noise, and I couldn't read or watch tv, or talk on the phone. It was hard to eat and my thinking was a little off.

At first they told me I had profound hypothyroidism. The only medication I was given in the beginning was thyroid hormones. HE was diagnosed after I was severely sick for 6 months.

For my initial treatment of HE I was given 60 mg prednisone and with that I could walk better, think better, sit up for longer. I could swallow and chew better. My episodes improved and my husband said he got his wife back. But I still felt sick.

They tried switching around my thyroid hormones. T-4 was a trigger. Once we lowered the prednisone and added Cellcept my symptoms improved. My moments of clarity lengthened. The severity of episodes lessened. Later we dropped the Cellcept and added Naltrexone. This drug has helped me heal.

Today, my capacity in all things is limited. I work from home typing up insurance policies. This is a good job for me. It is interesting because it is surprisingly involved but not taxing. I compare it to playing scrabble on line. I cannot drive because if I get startled I cannot react reasonably. I haven't applied for disability because my husband works.

Jennifer (age at diagnosis: 48)

as told by her husband, Jim

My name is Jim and my wife, who suffers from HE, is unable to write. In fact, she still suffers greatly from impairment of her motor skills, understanding, reasoning and memory that was brought on by this rare disease, so I will begin telling our story that began 11 years ago this September 2013.

First though, my wife and I have been married 24 years at the time of onset and we met in San Francisco. By the way, my wife is Chinese American, brought up in here in San Francisco. She speaks very little if any Chinese and you wouldn't know she was Chinese if you spoke with her on the phone. My wife was a receptionist for a Chiropractor in California for about 12 years before the illness began.

My wife, youngest daughter, and I have since moved to Tennessee. My wife was a stay at home mom just before her car accident which I will now explain.

We have three children (all born in California) and the only male was 20 years old when he was diagnosed with an aggressive Intermediate Lymphoma in his sinus cavity. Doctors told us he had a 50/50 chance of survival. He had a bone marrow transplant which saved his life, and he has been in remission for 14 years now.

Right after that my wife and youngest daughter were in a serious car accident in our small Tennessee town and a pickup truck going 60 mph hit them broadside. Both were taken to the hospital with very serious injuries. My wife had all left side bones broken including all ribs, collar bone, pelvis, low back and a punctured lung, but by the grace of God they both survived. We applied for Social Security disability but were denied until my wife was diagnosed with HE shortly thereafter, and she has been on SS to this day (July 2013).

About two years after the accident my wife woke up one day and things were opposites to her: cats were barking...she said she was sitting when she was actually standing…she made herself 2 cups of coffee at the same time when she only has one cup every morning…she had difficulty walking…and just generally acting strangely. I drove her to the hospital thinking she had a stroke. She spent several days and had many tests in the hospital, but the doctors in this small-town Tennessee hospital came to no conclusion. They then released her to my surprise.

We came home for not more than a couple of hours and my wife went into convulsions, so I called 911 and they sent her to another hospital on the other side of town, where later that night they transferred her to UT Medical Center in Knoxville.

At this point my wife started to get worse. She became very confused, and her motor skills and reasoning were like that of a small child. I had to do everything for her - she was almost as helpless as a baby.

The doctors had done every known test and she had seen every specialist in the Hospital, in fact she had two neurologists that both had many years of service and still no one could give me a diagnosis. There would be groups of interns that would come in throughout the day asking questions but they wouldn't say much.

My wife also had MRI's, CT scans, numerous blood work-ups, ultra-sound of her thyroid and a spinal tap. All tests came up negative! It was very frustrating to say the least! I did tell the doctors that the day before her initial hospitalization we were shopping for carpet and at the warehouse was a very aggressive and pesky fly or mosquito that was just relentless and bothering us big time but unknown if it may have bit her - no bite marks were ever found. Nothing conclusive on that though.

The head neurologist spoke with me privately around the 15th day of her hospitalization at UT and told me they just couldn't pinpoint the issue, so he told me he would like to transfer my wife to a clinic of my choice. I decided to have her flown to Stanford Medical Center in California after spending a total of 18 days at UT.

Again, my wife went through multitudes of tests from a multitude of doctors at Stanford including a second spinal tap. One doctor wanted to do a brain biopsy but after further review I turned him down because it was too risky. He thought my wife had Creutzfeld Jacobs disease which in our terms is Mad Cow disease. It's a deadly disease - once diagnosed it kills! But thank God she didn't have that dreadful disease! Then the diagnosis came: 70% chance of HE is what the Stanford doctors told me.

Stanford doctors started my wife on a regimen of steroids and Levothyroxine at dosages I don't remember (dosage today is 50 mcg of Levo only). After that she began to slowly recover, very slowly- that was the best news ever. I will add that back in February 2013 my wife regressed, and the week before my wife had a blood work up from our family doctor and he changed her Levothyroxine dosage from 50mcg every day to ½ pill every day with no pills on the weekends. That's about the same time my wife began to regress, so then her doctor changed it back in hopes it she would improve but she has not. It's now July 2013. So whether this change in dosage had anything to do with this regression is unknown at this time.

We finally came back home to Tennessee from Stanford and my wife was still improving. She stayed on the steroids for about 6-8 months before the UT doctors took her off them. The only side effect that I remember from the steroids was my wife gained some weight and her face had swelled a bit.

My wife today has improved to about 65% of normal but still has many issues: memory, confusion, repeating herself constantly, reasoning problems, impaired motor skills including walking, eye/hand coordination, swallowing and some speech impairment to this day.

Over the past 10 years we did see our neurologist once every year and there would be periods of setbacks that would last for weeks but then bounce right back without steroids or any medications. But this past late winter 2013 she had a setback (dementia symptoms becoming worse) and to this day the symptoms have not improved. The neurologist wanted to try a 5 day course of 500 mg IV Steroids. I hated to put my wife through it but we decided to give it a try. The steroids had no effect, it only made my wife on edge. So, now we are going to a new endocrinologist and he suggested hormone injections which also had no effect. Now in September 2013 my wife has another issue: a racing mind, maybe like an anxiety of sorts, and it comes and goes throughout the day. I tried 10 mg Melatonin and 200 mg L-theanine several times a day and it seemed to help but not all the time. It was so bad one Sunday we went to the ER but all tests were negative.

So, back to the doctor again and he now has given us 50 mg Amitriptyline and 25 mg Hydroxyzine both two times a day which makes her very sleepy, but according to the doctor should wear off in a few days. If this doesn't work we are heading to Knoxville again.

My wife also had a CT scan of her brain in September 2013 but other than some normal atrophy it was negative. My wife will be 60 next year.

My wife also has an older sister that was diagnosed with Graves disease years ago. I don't know any details though! My wife's mother passed away of liver cancer at age 40.

As you can probably tell, this has changed my whole life and in fact I had to take early retirement because of my wife's illness. I was not ready to retire but I needed to, to be there for my wife full time! We were very blessed in that sense!

There are times when my wife understands what's going on but not really sure to what degree. Just before my wife's setback this year she usually dressed and used the bathroom by herself. But now I'm back to helping her get dressed and using the bathroom again. Since the onset she has always needed help walking and showering, taking meds, fixing meals- actually I've been doing all the cooking and cleaning to this day.

Of late, there's a new twist: I noticed that when we eat dinner my wife will fill her mouth full of food until her cheeks bulge, then gag or choke and spit it out. So now I have to watch for that. Every day is an adventure. My wife is more like my child than the wonderful woman I married 35 years ago. I just want my wife of old back!!

Hopefully there will be more research on this ugly illness in the future and find a cure!

I hope and pray this story is of some help to those who like me are looking for answers to these rare diseases and maybe even give some insight to the doctors who are looking into HE in more depth. One of my biggest concerns now is, is HE hereditary??

God's mercy and grace on all of us!

Louise (age at diagnosis: 49)

When life throws you a curve ball, the manner in which you tackle it can make or break relationships, friendships, work relationships and yourself. Speaking as the receiver of a very nasty curve ball back in October 2009, I can tell you that finding someone or something to blame is a waste of precious time and energy. Being brought up by devote Catholic parents I supposed I could have resorted to the usual cry of "It's all God's fault" or "Why me?" Nineteen months into this unusual curved ball I can truly say I must be made out of stern stuff especially coming from the Smith and Watson heritage, or going back another generation, even maybe Clutterbuck or McKenzie heritage.

What was the curved ball I received? Well it started like a stroke; I was in a staff Professional Learning Team meeting after school. I had had a sharp pain in the left shoulder and breast that had been niggling away throughout the day that intensified as the meeting progressed. One of the teachers asked me if I was okay to which I said "not really" and left the table and rushed to the ladies where I knew all was not okay, I only just made it! I vacated the ladies and rang my partner in life and crime and asked him to let our GP know I was coming straight there to the surgery where he had an appointment and to please not leave. I told the principal and staff I was heading off to the doctors attempting to make light of the situation and not alarm anyone.

Thinking that it, whatever it was, was not really that bad, I got in the car to drive the 16 kms in peak hour traffic to my GP's surgery. During the drive I lost the use and feeling of my left arm from the shoulder down. It felt like a dead heavy lump of timber and was equally as useless. The left side of my neck and face also began to lose all sense of feeling. I had to slap that side of my face during the last ten minutes of the trip to see if I had any feeling in it. A small but increasing sense of fear started to creep into my mind as I continued the drive to the surgery.

I had driven the damn route twice a day for more than four years and I must say it was the longest and slowest I'd ever driven it. I actually passed a Victorian Ambulance paramedics base and for a fleeting second wondered if I should pull in and ask them for assistance. Of course being the stoic, independent and possibly stupid but fortunately lucky person I am, I drove on to the GP's surgery. The longest thirty minutes I've ever driven. I can equate this drive to the three trips I've made to hospital when having my children and this one certainly tops the lot except for maybe the fact that I didn't drive through any roundabouts like when my daughter was insisting on making her way into this world and having a partner realizing he might just be the one delivering the baby in his father-in-law's old blue Mazda, something we can laugh about now nearly fifteen years later. So maybe as time goes by I too will look upon this trip in the same light and wonder how on earth I actually managed to get from the school to the surgery in one piece.

I walked into the GP's surgery and into his room only to be met by both my partner and GP standing up and in unison telling me that I look like s**t! Thanks fellas!

The GP asked me a few quick pertinent questions whilst ushering me down to the nurse's room where they have a portable EKG machine and anything that would assist them if I actually was having a heart attack or worse. The GP informed my partner and me that he was organizing an ambulance and I was going to hospital ASAP. Two of the other doctors from the practice also came to assess the situation and all agreed that the wisest thing to do was to go to hospital.

The ambulance arrived and once again I had to tell them all what had happened and I was given aspirin as a blood thinner just in case it was a Stroke. Then came the questions, had I had this pain before and of course I said "yes on Monday." They asked me what I did. My response was unexpected, I had got on the treadmill and tried to run it off or precipitate whatever was happening! Three doctors, the two ambulance officers and my partner all looked at me as if I was crazy. I was bundled out of the surgery and into the ambulance all the while still trying to organize my partner in dealing with two cars, three kids and his mum as well as getting back to the hospital. Well which hospital became a debate: the Epworth or the Austin. Austin won hands down as it was five minutes away and peak hour traffic. While on the way one of the paramedics inserted a cannula into my left hand as I was going to have blood taken and in preparation for anything else that was to come.

On arriving at the Austin I waited for quite some time before being seen, all the while more patients were arriving until administration put a halt on accepting any more ambulances as the ER couldn't cope. Lying on the trolley I was convinced that there were people much worse than me waiting to be seen, only to be told no I was of great concern. The Stroke specialist came and assessed me and set in motion tests, blood work, CAT scan, Nuclear X Rays, Doppler Ultra sound and chest X Rays. My partner managed to get into the ER and accompany me to all these and to help alleviate the waiting.

I have great admiration for the doctors and nurses who man the ER's. They certainly get pushed to their limits by patients and relatives who seem to forget their manners the moment they are admitted. My partner and my waiting time was alleviated by the ongoing conversation between two elderly gentlemen who had had the hearing aids removed and who were obviously neighbours and friends. We heard all about their ailments, their family, a dog and rescuing the dog from the pound, what it cost and the happy ending and the snoring! I must admit it helped keep my fear in check. Throughout the night and into the next day when I was admitted into the Stroke ward my partner and I had plenty of time to talk about what-if's! Late that evening as all the results came back they decided I could go home and see my GP ASAP. My husband stayed by my side the whole time ensuring I was supported, loved, kept amused and most importantly not alone.

At home I crawled into bed....

Thinking back I know my husband was s**t scared. He had to begin shouldering all the responsibilities I had been doing for forever. Little did he or the children realize how much I actually did do around the house, for each of them aside from working 60 to 70 hours a week at school. They always say if you want a job done give it to a busy person, that busy person was me. I never said NO, was always happy to oblige. Just maybe this lead to me blowing a poofer valve and having a migraneous stroke.

How things change! In the long sixteen months I have felt very alone. It appears everyone around me blames their bad moods, depression and anger, ails, inability to do stuff, lack of holidays and outbursts on my weird illness. Hashimoto's Encephalopathy is a weird and unusual thyroid auto immune disorder. It gets major front row blame for a husband's inability to travel for work. For an inability to apply for promotions that would take us away from Melbourne to exotic places like Africa, Mongolia, South America, places where medical help is not all that great. An inability to fulfill all the plans and holiday dreams they had made upon returning from Ireland. Ultimately for all the big and small things I did that made our lives run smoothly before I got ill that have now fallen onto his broad shoulders.

A teenage daughter has had to have a safety network set up for her at school so that if this illness I have did lead to my death she would have a group of caring, knowledgeable adults around her ready and able to support and assist her in her times of great need. Surprisingly this network has been well used over the months not because of my illness but because of my 23 year old son's lapse into severe depression and suicidal attempts. A huge lesson in life for a fourteen year old to experience, learn about and eventually see the sunshine through some very grim, dank dark days, months, nearly a year!

A young adult son suffering from severe depression and has to be let hit rock bottom and ask for help. How can any parent watch their child suffer and yet know they can only help by not intervening? Did my illness and uselessness get a pounding over this! It was laid squarely at my feet by my son. I suppose he had to blame someone or something before he decided to dig himself out from all the s**t he had buried himself under. Or as his dad said 'unpack the suitcase he'd been carrying around with him for years!' My son is a very lively young man who could have first and foremost ended up in a box in the ground by his own hand, stupidity, selfishness, egotistical self-wallowing. He is a very lucky young man because his parents and siblings seem to have an endless amount of common sense and love. He did try to wreck his relationship with family and friends but with the right help from our fantastic GP and a councillor he has begun to rebuild and reforge relationships and enjoy life. Nothing is hidden or ignored. It's true that a simple text R U ok? can work wonders. I badgered him for days, weeks, months and one day he rang home and just said "Mum I love you!"

From that moment on I knew he'd be ok but that he still had a long way to go. He has worked, played, re forged friendships and found out who are his true friends. Now days I just sent a text that says, Are you safe? And his response is usually ☺

My eldest son, his fiancé and cat all moved back home so they could save a deposit for their home. Six adults and a cat have certainly strained the house, water, food and electricity. Showers in the morning have become a race for the hot water. Still we are fortunate the house was big enough to accommodate everyone. The kids moving home has allowed my husband to travel for work not necessarily with an easy mind or heart but with the knowledge there are two extra adults at home.

You hear a lot about dysfunctional families and as I write this I see how easy it is for a family who seem to be relatively sound all of a sudden start to pull in different direction. Is this how we all deal with the possibility of death happening upon someone we love? Not running away, but immersing ourselves in other things hoping that when you pop up for air my unexplainable illness was all a dream, never happened, is a figment of our family's imagination. Who Knows!

In sixteen months I have had MRI's, CAT scans, x rays, Doppler Ultra sound, Lumber puncture, ECG, seen a neurologist, rheumatologist, endocrinologist, infectious diseases specialist and an Internist. I have given litres of blood for all sorts of weird and wonderful test. One sane piece of advice and insistence from my GP was I had to see a councillor. This person has been amazed at how well I have coped and remained positive and optimistic. There are times when I wonder whether I can remain in this positive and optimistic frame of mind.

Two years passed by and I had a new battle on my hands beside my health. I needed to get back to work. I commenced work two mornings a week, strange I feel like a stranger looking in. The workplace has changes during my absence. Colleagues don't appear to want to know too much about my illness, I think they are thankful it didn't happen to them and then the Catholic guilt thing kicks in.... It's my illness, my life, my family and my career.

My perspective has changed; living and staying alive has become the most important thing in my life. Doing whatever it takes to get well and get my life back. I know there will be a new normal but that new normal doesn't have to be too far away from what was normal pre Hashimoto's Encephalopathy.

Husband, lover, friend, partner, pain in the arse, bread winner, carer, taxi driver deserves all the love I can give, for without his obnoxious bullying, nagging, high expectations, tantrums, you name it he's turned it on, I would not be where I am today. Love what is it? It is all the above and more. It is the being there when the chips are down, the shouldering the load because the other cannot, it's doing all of the little things without being asked, it's the just being present when the other is god awful pain that will not subside and nothing appears to make it go away. It is the tolerating Darth Vader beside you in bed and the laughter and giggles at the enormity of it all. It is the holding, cuddling being!

Sex, well that's been hit and miss. Amazing how much you want it when you're ill and you physically cannot have it! It's like being a kid in the lolly shop without any money. Is it the be all and end all of a relationship? Only if you want it to be. Boy did we have to get creative. We should have dug out our copies of "The Joy of Sex" and the "Karma sutra" they might have given us extra alternatives and ideas. Drugs turn your libido off and what a pain that is especially when Hashimoto's Encephalopathy has already caused parts of the body to be numb to touch, feelings, temperature and sensations all messed up. It's like someone has removed the spark plug and re wired the brain, something is haywire and you don't know how to fix it, that is if it can be fixed, whether it just the drugs or the illness.

You are definitely like a kid in a lolly shop without any money. Oh how you wish the switch would turn on and everything return to normal. Alas life can be a bitch and this is one symptom that has certainly stretched and strained pulled us together and wrenched us to the core of our being. Life is too short to worry about little things. There are much bigger things to think about. Love is the underlying essence of a relationship, friendship is its cement. Thank god for our friendship.

Well what now?

Young adults have bought and begun refurbishing their first home. They have moved out and taken the cat! They have celebrated their engagement and are now planning their wedding for 2012. Thank goodness we are parents of the groom. Young adult son has begun to stand on his own two feet, get himself out of debt, hold down two jobs, enroll and attend a hospitality course that credits his skills in the industry. He is having many wins on many fronts. University is on hold until he has enough fire in his belly to pursue it, which is in his hands. Foremost he is happy and loves life. My daughter just has to be herself, enjoy being a teenager and do all the things teenagers do within reason.

For my husband and me, life is too short to worry about the past two years. We have heaps to do, places to visit, friends and family to catch up with and a cabin to chill out at when we want to. Maybe that's what getting ill was all about. Finding out what really is important in life. I can't say Hashimoto's Encephalopathy hasn't changed me, it has. There are still things I can't do or is not happening for me and annoys the hell out of me, but so what! There is a lot more I can do, and do well and will continue to try to do each day, each week, each month.

My husband, he's changed too! He's been beaten around, tossed upside down and just about lost someone he's been with for forever. So of course he's changed. He smarts when things don't go to plan. He explodes more often than before. He worries about stuff. He wouldn't be him if he didn't. The one thing I have never taken for granted through all these ups and downs is his love. There have been moments when the going was tough but he stuck it out. There have been times when I didn't think I could stick it out but he has made sure I have. That's Life, that's love and that's family.

If everything was simple life would be boring. Though for a little while now simple would do just fine. No curve balls wanted!

What have I got?

Hashimoto's Encephalopathy, migranial stroke with thyrotoxicosis. A mouthful, not curable, but treatable. Can I live with it, I don't have a choice! Will I let it rule my life? No Way! There is too much I would like to do, see and go, participate in. I have participated in the Pink Walk. I can ride my bike. Hot air balloon ride, Travel the Ghan have the energy and ability to keep up with my trim handsome husband now that he is by far fitter and more energetic than me. I so admire the way he has kept up with his fitness regime, mind his diet and stay positive. It hasn't been easy and he too could have easily given up on himself. He hasn't and for that I am truly thankful. His energy surprises and delights me. I hope in time I can keep up with him and hold my own, who knows.

Am I writing mindless drivel, to some maybe, but for those people who know me I don't think so. Why have I written about it, maybe to make sure that it hasn't been a figment of my imagination or that I was going mad? Maybe I am mad, I applied for admission for post grad studies at Melbourne Uni, I want to put my brain back into gear!

End note:- at time of going to print I completed a post graduate degree in TESOL from Melbourne University in 2012. I resigned from my primary teaching job and am now teaching adults English. It has been the best thing I have done, the hours I work are manageable, my work is full of laughter, living and love as is my home.

Julia

Until the fall of 2013, I was working very successfully as a research and development scientist, employed in a broad range of different industries and different capacities. In every position I have ever worked in, I was always the "go to" person when unexpected or catastrophic problems arose. Usually I turned a perceived problem around on its head, diving deep down into the underlying physical and chemical phenomena causing the problem, and resurfacing with patents and intellectual property for my employers. I was always a quick learner, allowing me to glide from one scientific discipline to another as needed to make any innovation that interested me.

I have always been athletic and had excellent balance and proprioception. I rowed varsity crew my freshman year at Harvard. I was a talented rock climber and mountaineer. At age 49 I started learning to ice skate, took up ice dancing, and was mastering silver level dances by age 51.

Then I had my baseline colonoscopy and my world came crumbling down. That was September 18, 2013. The problem was not my colonoscopy per se, but the various insults to my system involved in the prep, and some medical and pharmaceutical mishaps, that individually or in combination caused my HE to flare up.

Looking back on it, I think I may have had HE since the age of 42. During that year, 2002, I had a period of several months of listlessness, when I felt glued to the couch. My blood pressure became very low and fluctuated a lot during the day. Eventually I convinced my GP to start me on Synthroid, even though I was on still within the low end of normal for TSH. Within days, I bounded up off the couch and felt like myself again. Over the ensuing nine years, I had several other occasions when I would become a couch potato for weeks or months due to general lethargy, usually accompanied with significant bladder irritation. I took to wearing dresses all the time, because even the pressure of the lightest, most elastic trousers would irritate my bladder and urethra. I went to numerous urologists and had batteries of tests and lots of imaging, but no problem with my urinary tract could be found. Each of the bouts of lethargy and bladder pain would eventually resolve themselves.

Over the course of the year 2013, in addition to a bad bout of lethargy/UT pain, I noticed that I wasn't able to tolerate exercise under certain conditions. Whereas five years earlier I was rock climbing in the canyons of Death Valley, in 2013 I became unable to take even a moderate hike if the temperature outside was above about 70 F. I could still skate for two hours straight, but as soon as I got off the ice I would collapse in exhaustion and be bed ridden for many hours, or even a full day. Once when I got off the ice, I felt a dizziness and disorientation beyond exhaustion and almost asked my partner to come drive me home.

I had one odd incident a month or so before my colonoscopy. I found myself sitting at my desk, night had fallen, and the building was empty. I had no memory of what had happened since mid-afternoon. The next day my supervisor drew me aside and asked what had happened. I had no idea what he meant. Then he recounted that I had been called into the factory to consult with him and two manufacturing engineers, which I vaguely remembered. What I had no memory of is that while I started speaking normally, my speech rapidly began to slur, the engineers became rather alarmed, and my supervisor then led me back to my office because he said he didn't want me to embarrass myself further. I asked the engineers about it later, and they said it was as if I had become rapidly intoxicated in a matter of minutes, right before their eyes. I chalked it up to low blood sugar. Hah!

My colonoscopy preparation was MoviPrep, the main active ingredient of which is ethylene glycol, an atypical alcohol. Basically ethylene glycol poisons a person, and the body responds with a giant purge. I was trembling and weak by the time I was "prepared." During my colonoscopy, a small precancerous patch was found and removed, which made the procedure last longer than usual, and I experienced a lot of pain and never "went out" to the physician's satisfaction. He therefore administered four times the usual dosage of intravenous anesthesia during the course of the procedure. The active ingredients were a common cocktail of an opioid and a benzodiazepine.

After the procedure, I never seemed to recover. I experienced severe bladder and stomach pain and felt weak and lethargic. After several days I called the physician who had performed the procedure. He had come across as communicative and kind while the procedure was going as normal. But now that I was responding in a way that was not on his script, his amiable manner dropped like a lead curtain. He half yelled at me "There is nothing more I can do for you!"

This was the first in a round of unpleasant experiences with physicians who just didn't want to deal with anything that is unfamiliar to them, whose reaction to having no ready answer or immediate diagnosis, was to become angry at me, and even blame me. (Don't get me wrong; I have had excellent care from many thoughtful, open-minded physicians in my life, physicians who really took the time to listen and would treat me like an intelligent human who knows her own body. However, this was almost never by accident. I almost always had to search very hard to find such physicians, usually through referrals of other physicians who were my personal friends. The first neurologist to diagnose me with HE is an exception to my general experience, in that he is truly excellent and I came across him by accident, not personal referral.)

So I went to urgent care with my bladder and stomach pain and complaint of fatigue, and later to a doctor of internal medicine, in the same facility where I had my colonoscopy. I was tested for infection and inflammation, and had an ultrasound taken of my abdominal organs; the only thing found was antibodies to Pylori. The internist wanted to put me on a standard triple therapy for this, which consisted of two different prescription oral antibiotics, a proton pump inhibitor, and over-the-counter bismuth. However, there was a string of miscommunications between the physician's office, my pharmacy, and my insurance company. I recall receiving at least five telephone calls from the pharmacy that day, to the effect that my insurance wouldn't cover my physician's first choice of medication so that the physician would have to change to a second choice, and then a third, and then I lost track. When I finally showed up at the pharmacy, they had a prescription filled for only one antibiotic and for Omeprazole, and claimed that was all the physician wanted me to take. That is not what her records later showed. But I did not question the pharmacy, my thought being that since treatment of Pylori is so common, this did not require much scrutiny.

The antibiotic I began to take is metronidazole or Flagyl. It was developed way back in 1960, which I found reassuring;

surely both the short and long term effects were well-vetted. I do a little research on any new medication or dietary supplement I take. On Wikipedia and the other common web-based sources of medication information, the list of potential side-effects to metronidazole is terrifying. But so are the similar lists of side effects of nearly every medication, and so I had become inured and I was not alarmed, at least not until I began experiencing 70% of the worst side effects all at once. I'll jump ahead here and write that, now that I have begun to learn about the symptoms of HE, I find that many of the symptoms I had which could be interpreted as negative side effects of, or allergic reactions to, metronidazole are also symptoms of an acute flare up of HE. But the onset of my symptoms certainly was coincident with my starting on metronidazole/Flagyl.

I started taking the metronidazole/Flagyl on a Friday night. On Saturday night, I was dozing off to sleep when my partner snuck over to my bedside table to take a drink from my glass of water. I jolted awake in absolute terror, my heart racing, screaming uncontrollably, then I rapidly dissolving into weeping. Yet all the time, a part of my mind knew perfectly well that it was my beloved and trusted Larry there in the dim light. The technical term for what I experienced is over-responsive reflexes and hyper-vigilance. By Sunday, I was also experiencing confusion. I needed to shop in a grocery store that I have been frequenting for five years, to buy a list of items that I buy nearly weekly. But the thought of doing this suddenly seemed overwhelming. So

Larry drove me there and accompanied me through the store. Once in the store, I felt like a rabbit frozen in terror before an oncoming car. The lights of the store were painfully bright, the array of colors and shapes on the shelves was dizzying, a decision of even where to walk to get where I wanted dismayed me. I was literally staring at my feet on the tiles of the floor, and was terrified by the feeling that I had to decide on what tile to place my foot next. So many things that I could do so easily, so thoughtlessly just days before, were suddenly overwhelmingly difficult and terrifying. Then someone clinked two wine bottles together in front of me and at the sharp noise I leaped away screaming and burst into tears. Needless to say, no one else around me even blinked at the sound, but they gave me odd looks. By that night I was having the over-response reaction to visual stimulus, sounds, and even smells. I jumped out of my skin and cried when I caught a whiff from the cat box or from cleanser being used two rooms away from me.

The next morning, I felt a little better and managed to get my daughters off to school and myself off to work. It took me a long time to get there, however. I remember leaving for work, and then finding myself in the parking lot of my former employer, not at my current job. I couldn't remember how I had gotten there. I started out again for work, then drove right past my exit, and had to back track. When I got to work late for a meeting, I made a joke of my mishaps to my colleagues. I thought it was hysterically funny, and could hardly contain my laughter. Yet at the same time, a part of me realized this wasn't a comic matter, and that part of me registered the flicker of alarm in my colleagues' eyes. Throughout that Monday, my work, which I usually thoroughly enjoy, felt like torture. Normally I am on my feet most of the day, flitting between my laboratory, the clean room, the factory floor, conference rooms, my office; and I enjoy being on my feet. Colleagues used to tease me that I walked faster than anyone else in the building. But by that day, I had an aversion to doing anything that involved walking around. I became confused whenever I got up. I would find myself in an aisle suddenly fearful of the low sounds of the fans on the instruments around me, dismayed by the decision of where to next put my foot, and completely unable to recall what I had set out to do. I sat at my desk and typed up some experiments and put together a PowerPoint presentation on my computer, feeling fairly competent as long as I looked just at my screen and kept my hands resting on my keyboard. I went home early, got a lot of sleep, and felt somewhat better.

Tuesday morning I again drove to my former employer. I have no memory of getting there, or getting from there to my current job. Once I arrived at my desk, I was yet more overwhelmed by my work and felt a desperate need to get away from the source of disquieting indications that something was wrong and progressing to worse. The next thing I remember, was feeling surprised that I was in a grocery store 13 miles from my work place, with an obscene amount of chocolate in my shopping basket (all my life prior to that, I have had an unusually low attraction to sweets, and rather good self-control in my eating). Then suddenly I was back at my desk feeling a hot flash rise through my body, sweats breaking out on my back and neck, and my head feeling as though flames were blasting inside it. I remember slumping forward onto my desk. Then suddenly I was back in my home looking at my pile of chocolate bars in confusion and terror. It was as though I'd wake up again and again in different places throughout the day. I began to weep, and started to try to call the physician who had prescribed the metronidazole. It took forever. I could remember her name, I could use my laptop to find her number on the internet, I could recite all the side effects of metronidazole that I was experiencing using the correct terminology, but it took me countless attempts before I could enter accurately the seven digit number from my computer screen into my phone.

The physician was very concerned and insisted that my partner come home to be with me immediately. She asked that he call her back when he was with me, and instructed me to take no more metronidazole. When he called, she suggested Larry take me to the ER or to urgent care, but I irrationally refused, because I wanted to be home when my daughters would return from school. Finally she agreed to give me an appointment with her the next morning, with the caveat that if I got worse I should go to the ER.

That evening I was out of my mind and I knew it. I couldn't stop talking. Whatever came to my thoughts, I spoke. Part of me knew I should be editing myself, so as not to scare my children or hurt Larry, but I couldn't stop the flow of words. The smallest mote would set me off on an emotional rollercoaster. Something as small as a change in the expression of Larry's eye would catapult me from a conversation on the couch to a crouching position in the corner of the bathroom floor, where I would weep uncontrollably. But a moment later, I would hear my daughter say something that could be construed as a double entendre, and I would be laughing hysterically, really and truly delighted, and yet terrified.

We got the girls to bed, and I tried to go to sleep, but couldn't because I was very scared and my head was beginning to ache. I felt a painful pressure building behind my eyes. I began to feel pain in my throat, as though there were large, hard walnuts growing in it, pressing against my wind pipe. The palate of my mouth began to swell until it was smooth, and to feel as though it were being squeezed in a hot vice. Finally around midnight I felt my eye lids swelling. Some small shred of critical thinking kept working in me through all this. That part of me knew that my symptoms were consistent with a severe allergic reaction. That part of me used my phone to take photos of my swollen face in the bathroom mirror and try to write down some measure of my conditions so that I could decide if they were getting better or worse through the course of an hour. Finally at 2 am I awoke Larry and he took me to the nearest ER. I wish with all my might that I would have asked him then to take me to the next nearest ER, which would have been Stanford Hospital. Instead I was admitted to a maze of dysfunction.

My eye lids were so swollen at that point that I had only a slit of visual field and my left eye seemed to have a shrinking tunnel imposed on the slit. I could barely walk with help. I had almost no control of my limbs. I couldn't remember my birthday. But the admitting nurse was unperturbed by my claim to be having a severe allergic reaction. She was impatient with my feeble attempts to sign the admitting paperwork, and rolled her eyes when I couldn't lift my arm for her to put on the hospital ID band. Then she put me in a room on a gurney and left me for a long time. The pain in my head and palate and neck became unbearable and I began to try to call out for faster help. I knew I wanted an IV with epinephrine immediately. I knew they should do this for me. Then suddenly my legs began convulsing and it seemed as if the left side of my mouth was twisting off my face, and then at last someone was jamming an IV into the crook of my arm. A doctor pulled back one of my eyelids and shone a bright light into my pupil. I immediately projectile vomited, fortunately managing to spray the admitting nurse, who was then busily chirping at the alarmed doctor that "she wasn't at all like this when she first came in". A part of me was incoherent with pain and fear, and a part of me was laughing hysterically when she complained of the vomit on her smock. A part of me knew I should just tell them my headache was a 10 out of 10, but another part of me couldn't stop from trying to tell them that my experience of the pain wasn't linear; it was exponential. And then I couldn't stop myself from going on to scream out the difference between an exponential and an asymptotic function. No one seemed to understand the purport of this. So I switched to French, to no avail.

Not unsurprisingly, when I eventually got my records, I found the ER doctor had described me as "possibly the strangest women he had ever seen". He also wrote that he had found through an internet search that recently I had been seen for depression at Stanford Hospital Psychiatry. That was completely untrue. I later learned that it was probably impossible, because that hospital and Stanford do not even share the same computer database and network. Yet I think what he wrote biased my later interactions with doctors at that first hospital where I was admitted to the ER.

Through my IV port I was given opiates for the pain, I was given a benzodiazepines for the convulsions, I was given an anti-nausea medication, and I was given something else to bring down my blood pressure, which was 200/100 (my blood pressure usually has been on the low end of normal). They couldn't get me still enough to take a CT scan. Finally someone thought to inject me with Benadryl to try to sedate me and stop the vomiting, and my world suddenly got quiet. The pain lessened just enough for me to lose consciousness. I awoke projectile vomiting in the CT scanner and drenching myself in my own urine as my body convulsed. Fortunately the scan had just completed. There was no bleeding. I hadn't had a stroke.

Nonetheless, I was admitted to the Stroke Unit, for lack of a better idea of where to put me. From there, for the next three days, every three hours I would call the nurse for more Benadryl as I felt the burning vice begin to clamp again on my palate and the mounting pressure in my throat and behind my eyes made me desperate with pain. I was urged to take opiates and benzodiazepines. But they only dulled the pain, they didn't really help. I remember in the middle of one night a nurse standing terrified over me as he finally injected me with the Benadryl I had been begging for over the previous hour. I remember his look of amazement as he watched the swelling of my left eye lid begin to shrink within a minute of the injection.

In the morning a hospitalist came and explained that he was a doctor trained especially to coordinate my hospital care. I had read and heard about the rise of this specialty, and from a distance had thought it seemed like a very good idea. He started out with a perfect bedside manner, serious, sympathetic, rational and confident. He convinced me to allow him to perform a lumbar puncture to extract spinal fluid. He convinced me to accept benzodiazepine to relax me for the procedure. But he wouldn't change my orders so that I could have more Benadryl, and he wouldn't allow that I had probably had an allergic reaction to the metronidazole. As more and more tests came back showing nothing abnormal, as he was called again and again because I was demanding more Benadryl and sooner than his orders permitted, his manner began to slip. On the second day, as I continued to ask questions and to bring up my ideas of what I thought was wrong with me, he finally snapped at me "you're above my pay grade". I was taken aback. I wasn't sure what he meant at the time. By the end of another day, when he repeated it while rolling his eyes, I realized it was his way of calling me a hysterical woman in need of psychiatric medications to control my imaginary ailment.

But in that intervening day, I met a very fine, very bright neurologist. He came first to my roommate, a Catholic nun who had had a stroke. He asked her a few questions and then told her he was an atheist and recounted what had lead him to reject the Christian religion in which he was raised. If she reacted, it was inaudible to me. Then he came to me, and asked the standard sort of preliminary questions about what day it was, did I understand why I was there, and what I do for work. As soon as I mentioned that I used lasers to measure greenhouse gasses his tone became belligerent, he crossed his arms, and demanded to know what could be done about global warming. This is a question that easily makes me quite passionate, and I gave my opinion and launched into my supporting arguments. The more I talked the more he smiled, and then he told me he was confident I had not been significantly impaired by whatever had gone on in the ER and that I probably hadn't had a stroke. He recommenced questioning me, casting a broad net over every detail of my health history, and that of my genetic relations. He told me he would return to me the following morning.

As it happened, when he returned I was experiencing a bout of emotional volatility, crying to my favorite nurse about my terror, then switching suddenly to laughing when her face so visibly showed her effort to hide her bewilderment at me. He listened from the side and then stepped forward to tell me I was right to be frightened, and that for two reasons it was to be expected that I would be emotionally volatile. First, I had been through a terrifying ordeal. Second, he hypothesized that I might have a condition that would actually generate emotional volatility. Then I first heard the words Hashimoto's Encephalopathy.

On the computer terminal beside my bed he brought up the MRI images of my brain. The hospitalist had told me the radiologist had declared my MRI to be completely normal. But the good neurologist pointed out that there were about 30 bright spots (technically "foci of increased signal in the T2 weighted axial image") scattered throughout my white matter, that there were some points of subtle narrowing in the blood vessels in the virtual 3D images of my MR angiogram, and that I had an odd 6mm hole in my brain (technically "a T1 dark lesion seen within the left parietal lobe white matter"). He said that it looked like the brain of an 80 year old, or one who had smoked a lot of marijuana or used a lot of ecstasy for a long time, none of which described me. He went through a list of test results (that the hospitalist had declared completely normal) and said that while technically normal, several were at the high or low extremes of what is designated as normal, and that taken together with my symptoms, he felt this meant something. But one test value was definitely out of the normal range, which of course was a high level of anti-thyroid peroxidase (normal range: 0.00 to 8.99 IU/ml; mine: 57.3 IU/ml). Then as the coup de gras of his masterfully reassuring behavior, he gave me a bunch of printouts of the latest publications on HE and pseudo bulbar affect (also referred to more earthily as emotional incontinence) and handed control of the computer terminal over to me.

I was jubilant with my diagnosis. Anyone who has been through a horrifying medical emergency, has gone through multiple rounds of medical testing that turn up nothing, all the while feeling something is dreadfully wrong, will understand my reaction. Anyone who has been treated dismissively as a whining hysteric, with an imagination in overdrive, will understand what it means to be handed a stack of literature on a real disease. My favorite nurse had stayed to listen to all this, and had tears in her eyes in sympathy for my relief. The neurologist then said that he was inclined to start me on intravenous high dosage prednisone while I was still in the hospital, but first wanted to get the opinion of a rheumatologist, whom he warned me, in an offhand manner, was a grumpy old guy, but good. Oh, and by the way, he was leaving on a flight at midnight in order to attend a conference. I told him that sitting in that conference would be just so much ass-flattening, and he agreed. Obviously, my executive function that should have been censoring my speech was still impaired, but he didn't take it personally. The nurse lingered behind to tell me how fortunate the hospital was to have recruited so brilliant a neurologist just a few months prior. This turned out to be the red flag that I later recognized signaled that problems could lie ahead.

In the morning, a rheumatologist with a kindly, professorial air came and spoke with me for an hour and examined my hands and feet and skin. He said that in his many, many years of practice he had never heard of HE, had not yet met the good neurologist, understood he was young and clever. Shortly after the rheumatologist left, the hospitalist dropped in to say that the rheumatologist was inclined to wait and watch me for a bit longer before taking any intervention. But he would not absolutely oppose immediate treatment with prednisone. He, the hospitalist, told me confidently that he agreed with the good neurologist's diagnosis and prescription for prednisone, so that was two doctors against one, and treatment would proceed. Many hours passed and nothing happened. Finally I walked out to where the hospitalist was sitting at a station at the center of the ward. Before he even raised his eyes to me, I perceived from his body language, with utter certainty, that an electric switch had been flipped. When I asked about starting the IV prednisone, he replied that it hadn't been ordered yet by the neurologist covering for the one who had left for the conference, and repeated that I was above his pay grade. I returned to my bed, and in the late afternoon, in walked the covering neurologist.

He let me know that he had 15 years more experience than the good neurologist, and he had never heard of HE. Then he asked me to tell him in my own words what had happened. I started in with my medical history, but he soon cut me short by observing that I was at a very stressful point in my life and asking if I hadn't started taking a lot of sleeping medication recently. I was bewildered. I started to correct him, rather meekly I thought, on what he had just told me about myself, when he cut me off again. Waving his hand in a gesture to encompass my body from head to toe he spat out, "Look at yourself! You're perfectly healthy! You're fine!"

I wasn't fine. Every three hours, like clockwork, my headache, throat pressure, and pain in my palate continued to return, my emotions continued to swing around violently, and I was afraid of what would happen if I couldn't have the IV Benadryl. But in that moment I became afraid of staying there. What if they stopped giving into my demands for Benadryl? The hospitalist said that I couldn't possibly be experiencing an allergic reaction since my symptoms continued to recur. He said that if I had recurring symptom of an allergic reaction after an initial improvement, then I was the first person in history to demonstrate this. The statement showed he was woefully un-informed. Suddenly a lot of points of dysfunction that I had been observing in the whole hospital coalesced into a pattern before me.

The hospitalist wanted to discharge me with prescriptions for a tricyclic anti-depressant and an oral benzodiazepine, but he had never brought in a psychiatrist to examine me. He denied I had experienced an allergic reaction, but had never brought in an allergist to evaluate me.

The nurses didn't get along and I was in the crossfire. One told me another was lazy and he would force her to get up from her chair. Over my objections, he undressed me for my shower, then called her to say I was getting cold waiting for her. Another one would slink into my room and use the toilet there, rather than the staff toilet. He was on the night shift and I awoke several times to find him standing in the dark, at the foot of my bed, munching apples. When I expressed my uneasiness about him to his female coworker on the shift she confirmed that he did strange things and alarmed other patients. Bitterly she said he was so old that he made work for everyone else. She would see to the matter. Yet there he was in my room again the next night. The head nurse of the day shift, when another nurse or a doctor was in the room, would use correct hygiene while injecting medication into my IV port. But when alone, she ignored my protests against her using my roommate's soiled food tray to hold the syringes and vials as she prepared my injections; she denied that she should put on gloves for the process; and she neglected to wipe my IV port with disinfectant before the injection.

The computer system for recording and controlling medication was unreliable. When I was in the ER an announcement over the PA system warned that in five minutes the system would be going down for 90 minutes of scheduled maintenance. The doctor working on me was very evidently uninformed; he swore and started yelling frantic orders to draw down all the medications he feared he might need for me and other patients in those 90 minutes of down time. The hospitalist gave orders (over my objections) for me to get benzodiazepine to help keep me still during my second MRI. It was given to me promptly after I returned from my MRI. To cap it all, the second MRI was intended to be done with and without contrast, but wasn't very useful because a different test sequence was run in the before-contrast measurements than in the after-contrast measurements.

So I concluded that I might be better off out of the hospital than in. At least I could be sure to have as much liquid Benadryl as I wanted. To make me more comfortable with my decision to bolt that crazy joint, the hospitalist walked in just then to say that the he agreed with the cover neurologist that I should not get IV prednisone, and that made three doctors against one. That was Friday. I slept that night in my own bed with a bottle of liquid Benadryl beside me.

The following Monday, I saw my excellent general practitioner of many years. He reviewed all the contradictory reports I brought him, listened to my account of everything, then said the only thing that was clear was that nothing was clear except that I should stay far, far away from metronidazole. He recommended that I start over with a neurologist at Stanford.

In the meantime, my affect had transformed from wild swings between tears and laughter to something that was eerily flat. My dysarthria continued, with my tongue to feeling as though it were too big for my mouth and my speech rhythm jarringly uniform, like an outdated science fiction movie rendering of a talking computer with a lisp. My daughter, in irritation, asked me to "please stop talking in that funny, fake voice". But I couldn't. I could only lose my wooden affect for a few minutes to respond with a burst of tears. I tried to go to work, catching a ride with a colleague, since I knew it wasn't safe for me to drive. But I was worse than useless. I was too confused to be productive, almost too weak to sit up in a chair, and was overcome with strange surges of sweats and chills. I fainted at my desk and was driven home before lunch time. I was so ashamed. I was hired and highly paid by my company to solve problems, not create them. Drama queens can be amusing, but, to my mind, never at work. I felt like I was coming off as a drama queen. I tried one more day to work, but the outcome was not substantially better. So I threw all my diminished resources at trying to get an appointment at Stanford Neurology Clinic ASAP.

People who have HE will probably know what I mean when I refer to my diminished resources. Many things that were triflingly easy in my past had become almost impossibly difficult, like figuring out which number I should dial to talk to someone versus the number to dial to send a Fax. Other things that seemed like they should be impossibly difficult if I couldn't dial a phone, were still easy for me. For example, I could read whole books of philosophy, history, and fiction, I could read scientific literature on HE, and I could assimilate the ideas and form clear synopses of what I had read. But I couldn't get through the process of ordering a new book using my existing account on Amazon.

The assortment of impaired and unimpaired function I have fits some sort of pattern. Most of it has the hallmark that I retain a lot of what would normally be considered high level function, and yet have lost what might be considered low level function associated with it. I used to imagine that my abilities were like my scientific training, and formed a sort of pyramid with a base of large area that tapered to a peak. I imagined that my highest attainments and functional abilities could exist only with the support of that solid foundation of lesser abilities. I could use thermodynamics only after I could use calculus, which in turn was preceded by basic math, and so on.

But I am finding now that is not the case for me. For example, I know my alphabet, I know how bookstores and libraries are organized, but I cannot pick out an author or a title even when I am standing in front of the very shelf containing the book that I want. Yet if someone gives me that book, even if it on something I consider complex, such as laser physics or the origin of anti-intellectualism in America, I can read it and write cogent essays about it. I can draw a diagram neatly explaining how a hybrid car works, but I cannot switch lanes while driving (don't worry, I have taken myself off the road). I can research prednisone, and later write down the reaction pathway used in its manufacture and list all the disorders it is used to treat, but it takes me four hours to obtain a prednisone refill and then I am exhausted and bedridden by the effort. I can type rapidly with the correct nine finger method, but I can't point and click with a computer mouse, and it takes me many, many attempts so use the touch screens that I am confronted with when trying to pay in nearly every store.

Twelve days after leaving the dysfunctional hospital I was at my appointment at Stanford. The neurologist there was very calm. He was perfectly familiar with my records and test results, and was familiar with HE and spent about an hour and a half with me.

I expressed my wish to start prednisone immediately, but he demurred. He said his prime objective was to do no harm, and he wanted more tests done to eliminate the possibility of Lyme disease, for instance, but he promised to call me the next day. I descended to the lab on the ground floor. Fortunately Larry was with me because there, I was confronted with those dratted arrows again, directing me where to queue up, and where to wait. I now find those things so intimidating that I think that without Larry's support I would have fled the lab before getting my blood drawn once again.

Much to my amusement, I was given a large plastic jug and some labels. I was supposed to collect every drop of my urine in the jar for 24 hours, keep the jar refrigerated, fill out the labels with the time I started and stopped urine collection, and then get the jar back to the lab in an ice chest within a few hours of completing collection. In my current state, nearly every step of this was a monumental undertaking with a high probability of mishap. Filling out labels? The word "time" was bracketed by a line above and a line below. Which line should I write on? Would it be better for me to use an am and pm designation assuming they would be using 12 hour clock, or should I use notation consistent with a 24 hour clock? I knew the ice chest was in the storage closet off the patio, but there was no way I would be brave enough to undertake the complexity of lifting several things off it, dragging it out, and then replacing the things that had been on top. Every time I had the urge to pee, I got into a do-loop of indecision. Should I first go get the jug out of the fridge and carry it to the bathroom, or should I pee in the cup and then carry the cup to the jug? I would rock back and forth from one foot to the other, immobilized by indecision. And what kind of slapstick comic had thought of asking me to pour multiple cups of urine into the neck of a jar that had a lid screwed over the opening every time I tried to do this? Needless to say, the first round of this exercise was rejected by the lab. I eventually succeeded in this marathon task with Larry's help and with a larger jug with a different lid.

The day after my appointment at Stanford, a nurse called to tell me a prescription had been sent to my pharmacy for oral prednisone. She rapidly instructed me that I was to start at 20 mg per day for a week, then ramp up by 10 mg in each succeeding week until my symptoms abated. I was also told I had a prescription for an ion pump inhibitor to alleviate possible stomach irritation from the prednisone, and I was told to take over-the-counter calcium and vitamin B supplements to maintain my bone density. Shortly, the pharmacy texted me that I had a prescription ready for pick-up, and with joyous excitement I began the slow meander, which I now practice as an alternative to walking, toward the pharmacy – the pharmacy with the dreadful arrows. Of course I was to be frustrated and disappointed. The pharmacy had no record of a prescription for prednisone. They had received a prescription for an expensive new ion pump inhibitor, but my insurance had turned it down. My wooden affect dropped and my tears returned as I tried again and again to phone Stanford Neurology and again and again reached their fax or completely random people who happened to have seven digit phone numbers. Before the pharmacy closed, I did have my prednisone and some over-the-counter antacid.

I had read that on oral prednisone, relief from HE, if it comes at all, will be felt within 3-10 days. On the evening of exactly the third day, I suddenly lifted my head from my book because of a surprising physical sensation. I felt as though I had somehow moved back into my own mind. I felt as though two transparent sheets, each with a meaningless assortment of splotches, had been overlaid and aligned and now revealed a coherent image. That image is the real me. I began to effuse my happiness to Larry, and he looked up, smiled, and said "your normal voice is back".

I have a follow-up appointment with the Stanford Neurologist in two weeks. Tomorrow morning I will have to decide whether or not to try to return to work. I feel I am myself again, but I am definitely still impaired. I still can't dial phone numbers, join a group on Facebook without Larry's help, keep track of time, drive. I took a short walk yesterday, and with only a few seconds of premonition to prepare myself, I was bathed in sweat and near-fainting on a planter on the sidewalk. I have developed a deep and urgent instinct that it is mission critical for me to stay calm and avoid physical exertion. My palate and throat still begin to hurt every 3-5 hours, and I continue to seek relief in Benadryl, despite the prednisone. I still slip into my wooden affect, or my pseudo bulbar affect a few times a day.

Through this ordeal, the horror of losing who "I" am, of losing my "self" has overwhelmed all other pain, and even made the fear of physical death seem dim. I feel like I am myself again, and yet I am different, impaired and with a whole new set of imperatives: Stay calm at all costs; keep a wide berth from over exertion. I feel certain I will have relapses of severe HE, I feel uncertain that I will ever be better than I am now, and uncertain I will every resume my career or dance and fly over the ice again. Larry and I talk late into the night about what it means to one's identity to lose abilities, to have personality changes. When does one become a different person? What happens to your commitments to a person when that person no longer seems to be there, although someone physically resembling them still breathes?

Ryan (age at diagnosis: 20)

So, I've decided to tell my story. Now, keep in mind that I'm not really the "story telling" type, so this particular story might have its dull moments. Bear with me though, because although it may be dull at times, it is a serious story, written about a very serious disease. This disease, as doctors would call it, is Hashimoto's Encephalopathy (HE); or to put it in layman's terms: a steroid responsive encephalopathy associated with thyroiditis.

Now, some of you may be reading this story because you have recently been diagnosed with HE, or some of you may have a loved one who has been diagnosed. That's why I've decided to share my journey, in hopes that I can help others through their battle with HE.

In September of 2010, I was riding back home from vacationing in Denver, CO where I had spent a week with my girlfriend and her family. My girlfriend's parents were driving us back home. We had had a wonderful trip, but were looking forward to getting home; we live in Iowa, so it was about a 10 hour drive. We had just stopped to grab a bite to eat at an Arby's, had gotten back in the car and were on our final stretch home. My girlfriend's mom and dad were laughing and talking while my girlfriend, Laine and I were relaxing in the backseat.

Since I missed out on a huge chunk of my story, I will share it with you through my girlfriend's perspective:

All of a sudden, I look over at Ryan and notice he's become completely stiff, his arms and legs were straight out and he was unresponsive, his eyes had rolled back into his head and he was not coming around. My dad quickly pulled over and we called 911. I was petrified. I had no idea what was going on with him. We had been dating for three years now and I was fully aware that Ryan was healthy as a horse...he hardly ever even got a cold. The only odd thing that I'd seen from him lately was some mild hand shaking when he'd hold a fork or spoon.

Thankfully, my mom is an RN and was able to somewhat fill me in on what she thought was going on. Ryan was having a grand mal seizure (later we would find out that this wasn't true, because you come out of grand mal seizures, and he wasn't coming out of this). The ambulance got there and took Ryan to a local small town hospital in Harlen, Iowa. The doctors there had no idea what was wrong with him.

They loaded him full of valium trying to get him out of his seizure-like state. When I was finally able to see him, he was lying in a bed, whipping his arms and legs around, still unresponsive.

Ryan was then life flighted to Children's Hospital and Medical Center in Omaha, Nebraska. Once there, they intubated him (put a tube down his throat so a machine could breathe for him), and tried to bring him out of this "seizure" for three long days, until finally, after huge amounts of Prednisone (steroids), he came out of it.

We were all horrified. All we wanted was an answer as to what happened and what we could do to help him. The team of doctors in Omaha gave us our answer, Ryan was diagnosed with Hashimoto's Encephalopathy.

The doctors began to inform us that this disease is extremely rare and that it does not have a cure, or even a very specified treatment. This news was heartbreaking; Ryan was alive and that was enough for us, but there was no cure for HE, no specified treatment? What on Earth were we supposed to do to help him!!!!!"

Back to telling my own story now: While still in the hospital, I came around within the next week. I had to go through physical therapy to get my balance back; I also went through speech therapy. My brain had undergone a major trauma and it was difficult for me to remember anything.

I struggled for about six months after that. I was put on gradually decreasing amounts of steroids (starting with 60 mg per day and over time decreasing to none), and was also on Keppra (anti-seizure medication, 500 mg twice daily). They also put me on Levothyroxine to keep my thyroid in check (this dosage varied).

Once back in Iowa, we went to doctor's appointments, which mostly consisted of watching the doctor Google HE on the internet. These doctors hadn't seen this disease before; they knew very little about it and had no idea how to treat me. They all had somewhat of a "wait and see" or "it was a onetime fluke" attitude. They did however continue to check my blood and then decrease or increase my dosage of thyroid medication. They also slowly weaned me off the steroids and seizure medicine. We were led to believe that as long as my thyroid levels are good, I will be fine.

I went through a lot of struggles after my episode. My memory was very slow to come back and just everyday tasks proved to be more difficult for me. It's hard for me to describe; so here is another insight from my girlfriend, Laines' perspective:

Eventually, after about six months, Ryan seemed to be back to normal, he seemed just like he did before his episode. He was no longer on steroids, his thyroid was in check, and he had moved out on his own. I was living with him, he was going to college, and everything was great.

Then, after two years, the nightmare struck again. Now looking back, his mild hand tremors that began to increase gradually could no longer be written off as his thyroid being out of whack, and his one night episode of stroke-like symptoms could not be classified as a "deep sleep" he was coming out of. These were all signs, signs that his anti-thyroid antibodies were about to attack his brain...again.

I had just picked him up from a weekend away. I had gone back home to see family and he had gone to a weekend retreat. On our way to our apartment, we passed a new Hy-Vee and Ryan said he would like to go. Once inside, we started grocery shopping. I noticed when he picked up an orange that he could barely grip it. His hands were shaking badly, much worse than they were even two days before. He made a joke and I gently hit him across the chest, by the way he jumped you'd have thought I was trying to kill him.

We bought a few things and then headed to the car. Once on our way, Ryan was giving me directions back home (I could go to a place a thousand times and still not know my way around). We were laughing and eating some gummy worms (Ryan's favorite candy).

All of a sudden, Ryan got all stiff, his eyes rolled back into his head and I thought he was choking. However, I soon came to the horrifying realization that he wasn't choking, he was seizing, and he wasn't going to be coming out of it. I pulled into a gas station and called 911. Luckily, we were right across from the fire department so they got there quickly.

The EMT's pulled him from the car and hooked him up to the heart monitors and such. I told the EMT exactly what Ryan was diagnosed with two years previous and to my relief, instead of getting the "what the heck is this girl talking about" look that I normally receive when I tell people about HE, I heard, "You're kidding me! My sister was diagnosed with HE too!" In this moment I was shocked, not only because HE is EXTREMELY rare, but what are the chances of that happening!

Once in the ER, I felt the nightmare that we endured two years ago coming back...and it looked way too familiar. There we were again; waiting...waiting to see what the doctors would say. This relapse that he was having was a mirror image of the episode he had two years before. We knew what was going on with him; we now knew that with the high amounts of Prednisone he would likely come out of it. But what still haunted us was that we have no idea how to keep this from happening.

Will Ryan ever be able to drive? Will he ever be able to be by himself without us worrying he might have an episode with no one there to call for help? If he was unfortunate enough to not get this disease under control, would the brain damage just keep building up and eventually lead to irreversible dementia...or even psychosis?

These questions were all an undeniable yes and we were, and still are praying, that someone will figure this disease out. I was also extremely frustrated because we had been to the doctor not even a week before this, with Ryan shaking badly, and even with the doctors knowing what his symptoms were; he was not put back on steroids or seizure medication! I was wanting to trust the professionals, but it just seemed like they didn't have a clue and this was extremely frustrating. If they didn't know anything about his case then they shouldn't have taken it on…let alone led us to believe that everything was okay!

The hospital that Ryan had been going to for check-ups did not have the equipment needed for his care. Again, we were frustrated. We felt like they shouldn't have taken on his case knowing that they didn't have the equipment needed. In his case, Ryan has very little time to waste once he has an episode and the wasted time spent at this hospital was not appreciated.

Ryan was then sent to Mercy Hospital in Des Moines, Iowa. Since the doctors knew Ryan's medical history, they were able to bring him out of his seizure more quickly. However, they were forced to put him into a drug-induced coma and it took him quite a while to wake up from that. Ryan was in the hospital for about a week, after being intubated, having a spinal tap and waking up from his coma, he was able to come home.

The only new piece of information we learned was that his CSF (cerebral spinal fluid) showed a high level of protein, which was apparently common for HE sufferers. Also, his thyroid levels came back normal, whereas two years ago his TSH was through the roof. This confused us, because we had been led to believe that if his thyroid was in check, the disease was under control. Turns out, his antibodies were through the roof, which is more than likely what caused this attack.

Back to my story from my own perspective again: We are now back at home and I am trying to live each day to the fullest. Ever since my first attack, my life has been completely different. With me having this condition it has been extremely hard on not only me, but my loved ones as well. As of now, we have not found a doctor, neurologist, or endocrinologist that knows much (I personally think they know nothing at all) about this disease and so far no one has seemed the least bit interested.

Sure, all of them are surprised that I have HE and attempt to tell me information about it but it seems as though every medical professional we've seen has automatically been on edge when speaking with me about my disease. It's as though they don't know what to tell me and are intimidated and frustrated with the fact that unfortunately, they cannot help me. I hope that I will be able to find someone out there who actually knows about HE and can help ease my mind. I am praying that I don't have to live the rest of my life in fear of what could possibly happen to me because as of now, all I know is that HE could kill me. I am technically able to drive after six months of not having a seizure. Since the hand shaking and stroke-like symptoms have proven to be signs that another episode may be festering, I plan to not drive if those symptoms occur.

I am able to do daily tasks as usual and am not currently classified as disabled. I am hopeful that I will be able to find a medical professional who has taken an honest interest in this disease. Unfortunately, the medical bills from my hospital stays are totaling nearly $70,000 and that is a lot of money for a 22 year old to come up with! After my second episode, I had to cut my college classes and plan to start them up again this year. I am hopeful that I will be able to live my life free of stress regarding my disease someday. As of right now it is a major stressor on my life and I can only hope that sharing my story with others will help someone out there in some way.

Barbara (age at diagnosis: 43)

Approximately eight years ago I noticed ringing in my ear, and some dizziness. I was feeling really tired, and hadn't slept well for a couple nights. I went to see my doctor as a walk-in, and she ran some blood work, and scheduled me to come back in a couple of days.

I went to work the following evening. I worked in a locked down treatment center for teens, and I noticed that evening that the noise was overwhelming, and I kept having dizzy spells that made me need to sit down. That night when I went to chart, I had difficulty with focus, and my writing was very sloppy.

When I got off work it was raining, and while I was driving home my eyes kept jumping every time my wiper blades moved. I also felt some weakness in my right leg when I went upstairs to bed.

When I woke up the next day I felt weaker, and I was kind of limping. I went into the kitchen to make coffee, and realized I was standing, and staring at my microwave. I knew something was wrong.

I went to my doctor, who admitted me to the hospital. She thought I had a minor stroke. My issues only got worse. Eventually muscle jerking and tremors took over my whole body. I lost my ability to walk, focus, and talk.

While I was in the intensive care unit a new doctor was called in. They ruled out Huntington's, CJD, Mad Cow Disease, and Lou Gehrig's Disease. I had blood work, and MRI's. The rheumatologist came in, and I remember him saying, "Today is your lucky day, I'm gonna save your life." He diagnosed me with Sydenham's Chorea, and started high doses of steroids, antibiotics, and Vitamin B12. After a couple of days I was able to walk with a walker, and they started physical therapy. I was in the hospital for approximately a month.

A year later I was sick again, although not as severely as before. At that point I was diagnosed with lupus. I was put on immune suppressants, and when I felt really bad I was given oral steroids. After about 6 months I felt whole again. I had some ups and downs over the years, but nothing compared to before. I was able to work and had a good life. The ringing in my ears, and the vertigo never went away, but I was ok with that.

Then in November of 2010, I had a bad attack. All the old things, and a few new symptoms. My lupus diagnosis was removed, and the hunt for MS was on again. I was treated with high doses of IV steroids, then had another attack, and was treated again with high doses of steroids. MS was never found. What they did find was Hashimoto's Thyroiditis, and high TPO antibodies. I had been being treated for hypothyroidism since my first attack.

I was referred to Dr. Newmark at Kelsey, and 2 endocrinologists, and a rheumatologist agreed that I had Hashimoto's Encephalopathy in April 2011..I have been on 2000 mg a day of Cellcept since then, which has helped, but I want to feel like I did while in remission so I'm exploring IVIG.

Update: November 2013

My doctor admitted me to the hospital on Good Friday, and put in a jugular catheter, then started me on plasma exchange treatments. I took them until August 2013. I was prone to infections, and I got one around my catheter, so I had to have it removed. The doctor then started me on IVIG in September 2013 and I am currently still getting those treatments.

I want to say that I did much better on the plasma treatments. I had instant relief during the treatment and felt "normal" for weeks after. I personally recommend plasma over IVIG.

Lisa R (age at diagnosis: 38)

My Battle with HE started in May of 2009. Let me start off with letting you know that some of the information is based on things I've been told by my family. I have no memory of the first year of this disease. I worked in a call center and talking to customers all day and having angry customers would get to me from time to time, but when this first started I would go home hysterical crying. I would cry over everything and anything. I was fortunate to be diagnosed very quickly but again, the process of a diagnosis is something I do not remember. During the first year I was put in the hospital for steroid treatment and I insisted to my mom that I had lunch with President Obama that day and she said when she told me that was not possible I got so upset with her. I'm sure there are many other embarrassing moments like that. I can only imagine what I said to some of my customers. I went out on disability August of 2009.

So, now I'll talk about the stuff I do remember. One thing I am very thankful for is I've had great doctors through all of this and that is very important when dealing with a rare disease like this. My first neurologist admitted he had only seen a couple cases of HE but was so willing to research and I think he was excited to take on the challenge of my case. When I was in the hospital for a week having IVIG treatment, he came to see me one day and I was crying from being stuck in the hospital. He put his arm around me and comforted me. That to me was so much more important that how much he knew about this disease. Unfortunately he left his practice. Before he left he had started tapering me off the steroids and when I was completely off the steroids I had a horrible set back. I went to his office and saw a resident that had been taking his patients and she told me she had seen MANY cases of HE and didn't feel I needed to go back on the steroids. Needless to say, my mom and I were livid. This woman who was only a resident could not possibly have seen so many of cases when my previous doctor who had been practicing for many years had only seen a couple of cases.

A week later I went to the E.R. because of a bad case of hives. They put me on steroids for treatment and not only did the hives clear up but my HE symptoms improved as well. Needless to say – I found a new neurologist. He has been very helpful through this all too and unfortunately he has also left his practice. I am actually scheduled to see my new neurologist next week. Hoping he will be great too.

My symptoms of HE started with the severe depression and memory loss. Again, being I don't remember the first year, I can't say for myself how bad it got, but I'll speak about my symptoms from the times I remember. My biggest problems are the short term memory and concentration. I used to love to read books and could get through a novel in a few days. I found I can no longer concentrate on a magazine article much less a novel. I've been trying to improve that by reading easy books. Short stories and autobiographies. I can't even concentrate on tv series. That has improved and with the fall coming I am looking forward to getting into some of the series I've seen previews for. I can now get through a full movie as well without forgetting what the story was about.

I've also been very easily fatigued with HE In the beginning, I had a hard time sleeping at night and took the medication trazadone which helped a lot. I've always been the type of person that any sleeping medication had the opposite effect on me. So it was good to find something that actually worked and helped me sleep. I would sleep 14 hours or more and still be tired throughout the day. I would take my mom on our weekly trip to Walmart and could barely make it a few minutes without having to go sit in the car and wait for her. I would also have bad dizzy spells. The doctor thinks that was seizure activity.

There was one incident where I was at the gas station and went into pay for it and got really dizzy and passed out. It didn't take long to recover from that but was very tired and worn out after that. Another symptom I have is I've lost my sense of taste and smell. The doctors feel that is just a part of the damage to the brain. There is a positive to that though. I went from being 350lbs to being 175lbs. I am half the person I was before this disease, but unfortunately half the person I was mentally too. The doctors feel this may be permanent. While I am very happy about the weight loss, there are days I'd rather be fat and be able to taste my food. Parts of that have improved a tiny bit as well. I can tell there is a difference in taste with certain foods. If something is very salty of spicy, I can tell there is a difference but can't tell what it is. I was in the store recently and picked up a body spray and sprayed it on my wrist and could smell it!!!!!!!!! I could not tell the scent but I could tell it had a scent to it. I was so happy I had a huge smile on my face. I can only imagine what other customers were thinking about me walking around the store with my wrist to my nose and a big smile on my face.

I try to train my brain on this issue. I'll put pure sugar, lemon juice, salt and other strong tasted on my tongue and will smell different scents when I'm in a store I'll put different perfumes to my nose. All of these symptoms vary and sometimes will be bad and other times not so bad at all. But I never know what kind of day I'm going to have.

There are other things that have changed since having HE as well. I used to be a neat freak. I could not sit and relax or go to bed if there were clothes on the floor or furniture or something was out of place. I was always cleaning. Now my apartment is always a mess and it doesn't bother me a bit.

Things that I used to love to do don't appeal to me anymore. I used to love to spend summers in the pool. This year I may have been in there half a dozen times if that much.

I've also noticed my handwriting is horrible right now. I always had great penmanship and people would come to me to write stuff when they wanted it too look nice. Now I can barely read my own handwriting some days.

I used to paint crafts: Figurines, Christmas ornaments and things like that. I am just recently starting to try that again and am having a hard time keeping a steady hand and having it look good. I keep trying though and when I get one done it makes me happy.

I've been blessed to have friends and family that understand my disease. I moved in with my mom and dad about 12 years ago to help my mom who has bad arthritis and had her hips and knees replaced and doesn't drive. I have my own space upstairs in their house but it ended up being a great thing that I live here. My mom is my nurse, caregiver, pharmacist, and a lot of days my memory. We have a little joke that when she forgets something instead of Hashimoto's she has Hashimamas. But more than all that she has been my best friend.

I love my mom so much for everything she's always done for me but especially during this illness. I know I've changed in a lot of ways. I don't help her as much as should and I've become more self centered. I get mad at myself for this but can't seem to control it, but through it all she has put up with me and still loves me. I know I get on their nerves too because I am always hearing, "the answer is the same as the last time you asked that question".

So what is a day in my life like? Boring!!!!! I try to do things to help me improve. One thing I find helps a lot makes me look like a lazy bum I'm sure but I find playing games on the computer helps the brain a lot. I play word games, card games but hidden object games are the best for challenging my brain. I have gotten my energy back a bit and try to get some exercise in as much as I can. Taking the dogs for a walk or going for a bike ride, but living in the south during the summer, those activities are hard with the heat and humidity. I spend a lot of time on line too. Facebook is my social life right now. It's great getting back in touch with old college friends and keeping in touch with them and having good laughs about the good old days.

I am so glad this disease only affected my short term memory and not all the good memories from childhood and college. Facebook has also put me in touch with some great people on the HE page. It's nice to make new friends who know what I am going through and can understand and sympathize and mean it.

As far as treatments I've had that have helped and not helped: The steroids seem to have been the best. I was on cell-cept for a little while but that didn't help. I was on 60mg of prednisone to start with. I've been very slowly tapering off them again and am down to 2mg a day and am doing ok on that - not having the same setbacks as last time I tapered off them. I had the IVIG treatment. That did nothing for me except drive me crazy being stuck in the hospital for a week.

I know there will be some of you reading this who do not believe in God, but I have been a Christian all my life and do believe that God is helping me get through all of this. I'd like to share a song with you that I used to listen to all the time in college and about a year ago I heard it on a Christian radio station while driving and had to pull over I was crying so hard. It's a song I listen to when I'm having a rough day and it always makes me cry but also makes me feel better. It's called "Friend of a Wounded Heart" by Wayne Watson … here are lyrics from the song:

Smile –make them think you're happy
Lie–And say that things are fine
And hide that empty longing that you feel
Don't ever show it
Just keep your heart concealed
Why–Are the days so lonely
Where can a heart go free
And who will dry the tears that no one's seen
There must be someone
To share your silent dreams
Caught like a leaf in the wind
Lookin' for a friend–Where can you turn
Whisper the words of a prayer
–And you'll find Him there
Arms open wide–Love in His eyes
Jesus–He meets you where you are
Jesus–He heals your secret scars
All the love you're longing for is
Jesus–The friend of a wounded heart
Joy – comes like the morning
Hope—deepens as you grow

And peace beyond the reaches of your soul
Comes flowing through you
For love has made you whole

Tiffany (age at diagnosis: 28)

During the second week of March, 2010, as I was lying down for bed one night, my head started to spin. I had never experienced anything like it and it scared me to death.

When I got up to walk it off, my hands started to shake. After pacing for about 10 to 15 minutes, I felt maybe I was better enough to try to go to sleep. Thankfully I slept pretty well after that.

The next day I walked my usual two and a half miles to work. I arrived at the restaurant where I worked with enough time to sit and relax for a couple of minutes before we opened for the day.

As I sat there, I decided to call my friend and tell her about the episode from the night before. I broke down crying as I told her I felt there was something wrong with me. She told me I should go to the emergency room but I refused. I didn't have health insurance and I just didn't want any more debt.

The next few weeks were uneventful. There were a few times when I had the shakes but I didn't think anything of it. Then April 1st arrived. On this day, I was lying on the couch reading a book and suddenly I was waking up in the hospital, having had a seizure. After two nights in the hospital, they sent me home after running very few tests. They could not see anything wrong in the tests, so they sent me home with Keppra, which is a seizure medication. I was still having severe headaches.

After I had another seizure that sent me back to the hospital, I was finally diagnosed with Hashimoto's Encephalopathy. I was diagnosed by a female neurologist named Dr. Thomas, who wasn't even on my case. This time I was kept in the hospital for around four days. They performed more tests on me this time, including MRI's, EEG's, EKG's, numerous blood tests, a spinal tap, an ultrasound, etc. I can't remember a lot from this time as my head was pretty traumatized. I believe it was during this visit that I was in a coma and they had to revive me with a high dose of prednisone. Unfortunately, it was too much and I ended up with "roid rage" and accidentally punched a nurse, of which I have no recollection. After getting my dosage right and observing me for a few more days, I was released again.

My next visit was about four days later, on April 13th. My initial issue this time was not a seizure. I had eaten chicken tenders and potato wedges for dinner that night and almost as soon as I had finished eating, I had to throw up. While throwing up, I accidentally inhaled some of it. As I was going back into the living room to sit on the couch I began to have trouble breathing. Eventually it got so bad that I passed out, and according to my brother I turned blue.

After being rushed to the hospital and having a breathing tube shoved down my throat the wrong way, I had another seizure. According to my doctor my EEG test results showed some encephalopathy. My TPO levels were elevated all three times I went to the hospital. Another thing about this hospitalization is I had really bad hallucinations. I was seeing cars parked on the ceiling, the cold war was going on, I thought the tv shows I saw were based on my life and my family, and I even had thoughts that someone was out to kill me. This was definitely the worst visit and obviously the longest one.

When I was finally released from the hospital this time around, I was given Rispirdol for my psychosis along with Keppra and prednisone. I was also told to see a neurologist and endocrinologist every week for the next month. Eventually, after not having another episode, my visits were changed to twice a month.

The medication I was given worked well for me, at least for helping with my symptoms, especially since it's now been three years since my last seizure. I was taken off of Risperdal after a month. But I was on Prednisone and Keppra for a whole year and for most of it, I was miserable. The Keppra wasn't really the problem, it was the prednisone. It made me extremely hungry all the time, so I was constantly eating, and my whole body swelled up. I also became really depressed and moody and lazy. I have stretch marks on my body because of this time. But it worked, so I guess there is something to be said for that.

Today, I feel mostly like normal again. I do have occasional emotional mood swings and muscle twitches and extreme tightness at the back of my head, but for the most part I am doing well. I am able to drive and take care of my boyfriend and myself, and work. As long as I don't have a lot of stress on me, I am ok.

I must say that I have learned a lot about life from HE. I don't let things get to me as much and I have learned to appreciate things more. I have learned to accept this as a part of my life and I will not let it bring me down.

Helen (age at diagnosis: 47)

I will never forget the day my life changed.

It was Friday 7th December 2007, 8 days before my 48th birthday. I had not been feeling well, and had taken time off work. My husband Andrew and I left to pick up our granddaughter, Lily, from school. We were standing in the playground. I suddenly felt a strange feeling down the right side of my face. I shook my head and then came a feeling of paralysis and twitching around my mouth. Next came a strange sensation on the top of my head – going from the front to the back.

I turned to my husband and said, "I think I am having a stroke." I collapsed and that is all I remember.

Paramedics were called and I was taken to St. John's Hospital in Livingston. The next day, Saturday 8th December I was transferred to the Neurology Department of Edinburgh Western General Hospital.

The next part of My Story is a summary of my treatment, written by Dr. Robin Grant, Consultant Neurologist at Edinburgh Western General Hospital:

* * *

Mrs M was a 48 year old woman when she was admitted on 8 December following an episode of loss of consciousness whilst collecting her granddaughter from school. She had weakness of all of her limbs and there was jerking of the upper limbs. Her eyes rolled and the episode lasted about a minute. She then recovered but experienced a second episode whilst sitting down. It was during this that she bit her tongue. She was admitted to St John's Hospital and a CT brain scan was performed which was normal and she made a good recovery. A mini mental state examination test scored 25/30. Neurological examination was normal with no evidence of papilloedema. A number of blood tests were normal but her T4 was <5 and her thyroid stimulating hormone level was >90 with thyroid peroxidase antibodies significantly elevated. Her anti-nuclear antibody test was positive at 1/160 and double stranded DNA was negative. CSF was normal apart from an elevated protein at 1.12 g/L. Viral PCR was negative. CSF glucose was normal and CSF cytology was also unremarkable. Chest x-ray showed slightly over-inflated lungs but no other abnormality. MRI scan of the brain and MR venography was performed and this was normal.

Mrs M had been started on antibiotics and Aciclovir as well as steroids during her admission but when the antibody tests came back the likely diagnosis was one of an auto immune related encephalitis. It was also noted however that her vitamin Bl2 was low at 133 and her folate was low at 42. Intrinsic antibody tests were negative. She was commenced on Vitamin B12 and folate supplement. Her haemoglobin at that time showed an anaemia at 87 g/L.

Mrs M improved and was discharged on 14 December 2008. She was re-admitted on the 21 having felt non-specifically unwell with dizziness, nausea and vomiting and then she had a tonic-clonic seizure in the ambulance coming to hospital. This lasted at least 5 minutes and required Diazepam to terminate it. On arrival her Glasgow coma scale was 10/15 and she was hypothermic with a temperature of 35 deg C. Cardiovascular and respiratory examinations were unremarkable. Neurological examination showed symmetrically brisk reflexes and an up-going plantar on the left. She had signs of an encephalopathy which could have been postictal but related to the underlying problem. She was given intravenous Methylprednisolone and loaded with Phenytoin. Over the next 48 hours her conscious level improved significantly. LP demonstrated > 1 white blood cell but an elevated protein at 1.2 g/L. Cytology was negative. She was given intravenous Methylprednisolone for three days and then continued a course of oral steroids. EEG demonstrated asymmetry within the right temporal lobe but no frank seizure activity. Repeat tests for viral studies and CSF were negative. Ms M again improved while on the ward and a working diagnosis of Hashimoto's thyroiditis was made and her Phenytoin was changed to Lamotrigine. She did have some headaches and dizziness on standing and these persisted for some time but may in part have been due to her lumbar puncture. She was discharged home on 4 January but returned on 14 January having developed an itchy rash to the face and upper chest, likely to be related to one of her anticonvulsant medications (Lamotrigine/Phenytoin). She also complained of occasional myoclonic jerking and constant frontal throbbing headache. She was very anxious at that stage and was seen by the liaison psychiatry team who felt there were multiple triggers for generalized anxiety disorder. She recovered and was discharged on 26 January. I am glad to say seizures became controlled and her level of alertness and cognition improved but she had multiple other symptoms largely related to stress associated with the illness. She was started on Thyroxine during her hospital admission and anticonvulsant medication had been changed from Phenytoin/Lamotrigine to Keppra in view of her rash. She was on 20 mg of Prednisolone. Because of her anxiety she was seen by the neuropsychiatrists but she did not wish to start any other medication for anxiety/depression. The dose of steroid were gradually tapered over the next few months and by June she was taking Prednisolone 10 mg a day, Thyroxine 125 mcg per day, Levetericetain 1 g twice daily, and Omeprazole 40 mg. She had multiple symptoms consistent with panic but the seizures were controlled. She was seen by clinical psychology on 9 June who felt the anxiety was related to her fairly dramatic presentation with life-threatening illness on a background of some anxiety generally. We therefore did not consider that the anxiety was suggestive of active Hashimoto's but rather a response to her Hashimoto's. She continued to make good clinical progress and the steroid dose was cut down to 5 mg per day.

In December 2008 there seemed to be a clinical deterioration as she had been feeling nauseated and generally feeling unwell. She was re-admitted to the programmed investigation unit for re-investigation in February by which time she was taking Prednisolone 5 mg per day or on alternate days. She had some steroid associated proximal weakness and was feeling worried as her sister was going through a kidney transplant with a donor kidney from her other sister. Her MRI scan just showed cerebral changes associated with age but no focal changes in the temporal lobes. Kidney tests, blood sugar, liver function tests were all normal. Free T4 was within the normal range at 18, normal being 9—21 pmol/L. CSF protein was 0.71 g/L which was an improvement on previous testing. She had some treatment for her right painful shoulder and was reassured that there was no evidence of any active Hashimoto's. She had some vertiginous symptoms and was referred to one of the ENT surgeons. By February 2010 she was feeling generally better but had some intermittent flitting sensory symptoms in her face and there were some signs suggestive of steroid side effects. She had been doing Cooksey Cawthorne exercises for her vertigo which were felt to be benign positional vertigo. She did have some tremor but this seemed to be settling and she was under psychology management for her anxiety. By that time she was taking Prednisolone 5 mg a day, Kliovance for menopausal symptoms, Thyroxine 100 mcg, Leveteracetam 1.25 g twice daily, and Omeprazole 20 mg a day. There were no abnormal neurological signs on examining her. We cut back her Prednisolone to 5 mg alternate days and she was doing relaxation type exercises.

By February 2011 she was feeling generally better but there was very intermittent benign position vertigo and the liaison psychiatrist had suggested starting her on an SSRI (Citalopram) for her mood. Her Keppra had been cut back to 500 mg twice daily and there had been no further seizures. It is possible the Keppra might be contributing to her anxiety. We discontinued steroids and the plan was to gradually reduce and discontinue the Keppra and review her back in the clinic.

When I last reviewed her in the clinic on 7 July 2011 she had managed to come off Levetiracetam and has had no further seizures. There has been one episode of panic attack during an attempted MRI scan of the brain and she is much more confident. Her only medication is Thyroxine, Omeprazole, Kiiovance and Amitriptyline. There were no abnormal neurological findings. A CT scan of the internal auditory meati was performed at the request of the ENT department. She was unable to tolerate the MRI scan and I am glad to say that CT of the brain and internal auditory meati were normal. I saw her in the neurology clinic in July 2011.

Yours sincerely,

Dr R Grant

Consultant Neurologist

* * *

Has HE changed my life? Yes.

I was diagnosed with HE in December 2007 at the age of 47. Eight days before my 48th birthday. Prior to this I was in full time employment. I was a qualified Dental Nurse for nearly 30 years, 25 of those being employed by the National Health Service. It was a job I loved and miss very much.

I went through a horrific experience, as did my family.

I have struggled to get to where I am today. It has been very difficult. I know that without the expertise of Medical Staff and support from my family I would not have survived this. It does not just affect the individual, it also affects family and friends. The physical and psychological effects are tremendous, especially in my case.

I am unable to work. My employment was terminated due to ill health in 2010, and I was awarded ill health pension from the N.H.S.

I now suffer from:

- Panic, Anxiety Attacks
- Benign Paroxysmal Positional Vertigo
- Underactive Thyroid

- Tinnitus
- Balance Problems
- Bladder Problems
- Fatigue
- Memory Problems

I was told by my Neurologist to try and have a stress-free life! Easier said than done.

Daily tasks are limited and I tire easily. I cannot do things I used to do. I need a lot of sleep. I know I am not the same person I was, but I try and lead as normal a life as possible.

HE is a very rare and potentially deadly autoimmune disease.

There is no cure.

Kelly (age at diagnosis: 48)

I first developed severe symptoms of HE right after turning 42 (2006). All of a sudden my face went numb on the left side and I got extremely weak. I thought I was having a stroke. Prior to that I would sometimes get headaches with slurred speech and the inability to think, but I thought they were just weird migraines. At the time I had my first stroke-like episode I was a second grade teacher in an inner city school. It became very difficult to think. I felt that I was becoming someone I didn't know any more, and I didn't like it. I cried easily and could not control it.

My family/friends began to realize the severity of my problem because I was being taken from work by ambulance to the hospital on a number of occasions but they didn't understand. Even my doctors were confused.

As time went on my symptoms worsened, became more frequent, and varied. My vision would go in and out; I would feel like I was having a seizure or stroke. Sometimes I would almost pass out and be so lethargic. It was as if I was on drugs, or drunk. The muscles all over my body would twitch and cramp. I would fall asleep only to wake-up after an hour or so and not be able to return to sleep. I could not remember things, spell or talk correctly. And then I would gradually return to normal.

After seeing many different doctors, I finally received the diagnosis of HE in October 2013 from an Autoimmune Neurologist at the Mayo Clinic, in Rochester, MN, USA. (They call it autoimmune encephalopathy with thyroid antibodies.) Prior to the Mayo Clinic I had no diagnosis. I was told what it might be, Mitochondrial Disease, Narcolepsy, Herpes, menopause, stress, to name a few but never what it was. All they would say is, "You should be happy, it is not fatal. It will not kill you."

Before my diagnosis from Mayo, an optho-neurologist I had been seeing believed that I had HE. He had written my neurologist and primary care physician suggesting that I had HE but they refused to believe it could be HE. One doctor even suggested that I have my thyroid removed saying that it probably would solve my problems (I left her quickly). Another doctor from a large hospital in NYC saw me a few times then one day quit on me saying, "I don't know what you have but I can't help you."

In terms of my test results, most were normal. My MRI showed a small area of white matter signal abnormality in the high right frontal lobe region and a pituitary micro adenoma, and a sleep study showed an abnormal sleep architecture. Most of my blood tests, even some for mitochondrial disease came back within normal ranges. Only my anti-TPO AB is almost always > 1000 IU/ML, my Thyroid Recept.AB. is 1.92 IU/L. My TSH was at one time <.0001; it is currently 8.5100uIU/ml.

In terms of treatment, my initial treatment was 40 mg of oral prednisone for 2 weeks, tapering down by 5 mg every 5 days. After about 3 days on the prednisone I was feeling great. I hadn't felt that good in over 6 years! If I relapse, I will get corticosteroids via IV, at 1 gram a day. If I relapse more than three times in one year's time, the plan is to begin Cellcept..

HE impacts my daily life, and that of my family. There are days when I am having an episode that I cannot function correctly. Sometimes I am so vicious and extremely emotional. Other times I am so tired and weak. I am able to work but when I have an attack I am worthless. It takes everything out of me. I come home and fall asleep by 4 pm. A dictionary app on my phone helps me spell the simplest of words. My friends and family help with my daughter at times.

In a way, HE has changed my outlook on life. I cherish every day that I feel good. I thank God and my doctor who took a leap of faith and prescribed me the prednisone. But I am fearful that my memory is getting worse. I know that I forget a lot, which hurts. I hate myself when and I cannot remember events or words.

My emotional reaction to having HE is that it could be worse. Ask me on a bad day and I guarantee my response will be that I am tired of fighting and that I can't do it anymore but right now I feel great.

I am so grateful that I have had a few doctors that were willing to go out of their way to try and help me. Each one tried to solve the puzzle the best they could. They may not realize it but they kept me going even on my bleakest days. They listened to me and tried to find an answer. They aren't all the warm and fuzzy kind but I am fine with that. What I needed and wanted was an answer to what was happening to me. I want to thank those doctors for not giving up on me when so many had.

Diane (age at diagnosis: 54)

In 2000, my first symptoms started soon after my mother, my brother, and my mother-in-law passed away in a five month period. I also lost my job with Sears after working for the company for 24 years.

I had been experiencing some numbness in my feet, especially the left foot, and trouble walking down on any decline or standing still without holding on to anything. I went on to develop very poor balance. I went to my family doctor, Dr. Amani, and he put me on thyroid medication. Then, I fell at the doctor's office. I was walking and my legs didn't move but the body did (that still happens). I fracture a shoulder and had to wear a brace.

When I went to the orthopedic surgeon office, one of the doctors saw me walking and he wanted to see me. He told me I walk like I have MS and ataxia. I had all MRIs done on the neck and back. I saw a Dr. Schlenger and he did nerve tests on my legs and back and found irregularities.

That is when I started to see my first neurologist, Dr. Bukowy. He tested me for Lou Gehrig's disease and ordered all kinds of blood work. He ordered a MRI on my head and told me that it showed my head looked like an eighty year old women. I was only 52. He could not find out what was wrong with me. By this time, I was walking into walls because I couldn't stop and turn. My legs hurt all the time and if I would close my eyes or raise my arms I would fall or lose my balance. Motion also affected me. I was using a cane.

Then a miracle happened.

Dr. Bukowy went to California to hear Dr. Arnason talk about HE and MS. He was a doctor at the University of Chicago hospital. I had an appointment with Dr. Arnason in November of 2002. He took one look at me and told me I had HE. After the exam and lab work, my TSH4 was over 20,000 and counting. He said that damage had been done and I will always be like this.

He put me on prednisone and I gained over thirty pounds. I felt awful and was to see the doctor but I fell and broke my pelvic bone in my left leg. Two weeks in the hospital and finally I was able to see Dr. Arnason The prednisone was not helping and he put me on Cellcept. But after being on it for over a year, my TSH4 was still too high. Dr. Arnason than wanted me to have my Thyroid removed. It was removed in July of 2005. Dr. was amazed that my count didn't just go down rapidly. It took a year for it to get under 1000.

I lost some eye sight in my left eye, and my reflexes became extremely strong. I started to use a walker because I didn't trust my legs.

In 2006 I moved to Florida and started with a new neurologist, Dr. Hellman from the University of Florida. Dr. Arnason had recommended him. Dr Hellman was a memory doctor, and he was ok at first. Life was going well and I was doing really well with my walker. But I fell hard in July 2007 and fractured my right hip. I had surgery and needed rehab at home.

I was tested for osteoporosis and the result was surprising to all. It was a negative 5. I had no maintenance while I was on prednisone. I had a stroke in March 2008. It happened in the shower and I laid there for 7 hours until my husband came home from teaching. My speech was slurred with HE, and after the stroke it got worse.

I left Dr. Hellman in the summer of 2009. He wanted me to have Botox treatment on my legs. I know my legs are bad but I still need them strong to move. He said to me on a visit, "Why are you still coming to me?"

So my husband and I left the office and never went back. In the fall of 2009, I woke up and couldn't move my right arm and it was very painful. After many tests and shots and MRI's, the conclusion was that I needed neck surgery. Two of my discs in my neck were fractured.

Knock on wood; I have had no surgeries or hospitalization since 2009. My family doctor takes cares of me and monitors my counts closely. I still use my walker because I do not trust my legs. My legs get stiff when I sit or stand longer than an hour. I have problems with any kind of inclines. Also, my hands lock up when I am knitting or sewing. My fingers go together and I cannot separate them. It lasts for about 20 minutes. I have problems spelling simple words. I have to repeat things often or I get nervous about doing them, like walking to and from the car at a grocery store because of the decline. Stupid.

In December 2012, I dropped a glue stick and by accident I stepped on it. I got 3 fractures and a stress fracture from that dumb glue stick. It has been 5 months now and I still can't wear some of my SAS shoes.

The things that I have missed with this illness are:

- helping to care for my grandchildren - I can't hold them unless I am sitting;
- swimming - I can't figure out how to do this; I almost drown trying it;
- read a book - I can't remember what I have just read, so now I only read short stories.
- reading with others in a group - everyone reads faster than me and I can't catch up.

But, I still cook, clean, and garden. Ironing is a problem. I iron surrounded by cabinets otherwise I feel like I my going to fall forwards. Open areas scare me.

Drugs that I am taking now are:

- Clopidogrel – to prevent another stroke
- Mycophenolate – {cellcept}
- Atenolol – for heart
- Lorazepam – for nerves
- Levothyroxine – for thyroid
- Atorvastatin – cholesterol
- Calcium plus Vitamin D – Brittle bones

Michel (age at diagnosis: 50)

I had not been able to work since July of 2007, as I became disabled due to severe stress and anxiety and PTSD (which finally caught up with me after over 20-30 years!). This led to my having chest pains and having to be on numerous medications.

On Saturday, April 3rd, 2010, I got up around 7:30am and sat down to read the paper and drink my coffee; it was the day before Easter. My wife, Tanya, had been up for a little while and took the day off work to prepare ahead of time for Easter dinner. When I started to talk, I sounded very strange, like I'd had a stroke or something. It was extremely scary!!! My hands also started to flail and I had no strength in my legs either!

Our two oldest boys were home (ages 15 and 18) at the time and our youngest (age 10) had spent the night at his best buddies for a birthday/slumber party. Our oldest child and only daughter was at her home only 5 minutes away. I insisted that my wife call our daughter, Karah (age 24), to come over and pray for me. She also called our friend Victor, where our youngest had spent the night, and told him what was going on. She asked him to please bring Mikey home as soon as possible and join us all in prayer. We are very devout Christians who believe in the power of prayer and faith!

I was actually scared that I was going to die! I wanted to bless my wife and each one of my children before I passed away. After Karah got there, we started praying, my two oldest boys, Karah, my wife and I. Then I started my "final blessing" to my family.

I started with my wife, Tanya, then went down the line from oldest to youngest child, blessing them and encouraging them and telling them how proud I was of them! I really did think that I was going to die!!! When Victor got there with Mikey, he also brought his son Jeremiah and Mikey's other good friend, Garett. Victor is a mighty man of faith, who believes in the infinite power of a mighty and awesome God, so he also joined us in prayer, faith believing, as the Word of God says to do!!

My wife called the VA hospital (I'm a veteran of the US Marine Corp. and that is the only medical that I have) and they wanted her to take me to the nearest hospital emergency room by ambulance, but I refused, as I had no insurance and was concerned that we might lose "everything!" So, I had my wife take me to Mather VA Hospital, an hour away, which was the closest VA emergency room.

I was admitted and stayed there for several days. They ran numerous tests, and I was seen by a couple of neurologists. They couldn't find anything wrong with me. When the lady Neurologist told me, with my wife and all of my children in the room that "there was nothing neurologically wrong" I said "Then I'm leaving!"

It took my two giant, oldest sons and my wife to calm me down enough to agree to stay. After that, my wife gave word that that particular doctor wasn't to set foot in my room again.

I was discharged from the hospital with no answers of any kind and no real hope to find any. We were just told that I definitely did not have a stroke, even though all of my symptoms were "stroke-like."

In December of 2011 I was diagnosed with Hashimoto's Thyroiditis and was put on meds for it. My symptoms were still there, but maybe not quite as bad. Then, in August, 2012, my wife was watching an old episode of "House" and they threw out "Hashimoto's" as a possible diagnosis for their patient. She decided to google Hashimoto's, to see if there were any other diseases called Hashimoto's. She found a site with Hashimoto's Encephalopathy and listed there were about 24 symptoms of HE. I had 22 of them!

We sent the link to our daughter to print it out from work, as we don't have a printer, and took it to my next endocrinology appointment.

We gave it to his Endocrinologist at the Mather, California VA, and she read it and was quite impressed, as the information came from a very reputable site and she didn't even know how my wife found it. She then decided to admit me into the hospital the next day, August, 12, 2012, with Hashimoto's Encephalopathy.

We finally felt hope; something that we hadn't felt in 2 years, 4 months and 9 days. After 5 days in the hospital and beginning steroids, I started to speak normally again and the shaking had stopped. They sent me home with a diagnosis and treatment.

I started with 50 mg/day of prednisone, then weaned down slowly, as it gave me Type 2 Diabetes, which was a side effect that I definitely didn't want! When I would get down to about 25mg the symptoms would return, off and on; so I would have to go back to 40, and then I'd be right back to having Diabetes again.

This has definitely been a roller-coaster ride. Steroids have so many horrible side-effects that I have wondered if they are worth it. Steroids depleted my Testosterone so much so that I have no joy or excitement in anything at all. Another side-effect of the steroids is meanness.

I didn't realize that I was being so mean, but when my wife polled all four of our kids and asked them if they'd rather have Dad sick or mean, their reply was unanimously, "sick!" That was a huge wake-up call for me, as my children and wife mean more to me than ANYTHING!

So, I decided to do something about it and took it upon myself to slowly lower my dosage from the 25 that seemed to be my "stabilizer number," now down to 10mg/day as of today. During my last doctor's visit, on the 23rd of April, 2013, I told my doctor what I had been doing and she recommended weaning down by 1mg dosages, as 5mg would be too much at this point. So, I just got the 1mg in the mail and during the next several weeks, I plan to wean down further and hopefully it won't put me back in a wheelchair or a walker, but if it does, at least I won't be so mean to my family and my Testosterone levels will be back up (actually, I think that they already are starting to come back up), so that I can have some joy and excitement in my life!

In retrospect, I think that in my case the treatment of HE was worse than the disease itself! I know that this is an unusual disease and that not very many doctors know much about it, but until they find a better treatment, or God chooses to heal me, I am going to just keep putting one foot in front of the other and keep on going!

Misty

Before 2010: All my life I have had various medical issues including allergies, endometriosis, and preterm labor, tons of stressful events, and chronic colds and illnesses. Despite the illnesses, I have always been fiercely independent, highly intelligent, and a very hard worker. I traveled all over with just my child, worked 40-80 hours a week since I was 14, became a nurse, paid my own bills, and bought my own home all before 30 years of age. I liked to travel, go to the beach, read, advocate for children's causes, and play with the thousand-plus kids that attended the charity I worked for. In my job, I was often labeled a "super woman" by co-workers/bosses, I directed 100+ employees, founded children services programs, and devoted sometimes 16-20 hours a day to the organization. It seemed like I was unstoppable.

In February of 2010, I began to have unexplained progressive symptoms:

- Confusion/"Crazy" feelings
- Forgetfulness

- Light Sensitivity
- Floaters in my vision
- White Out Flashes
- Transient Vision loss in the right eye
- Swallowing Difficulties
- Speech Issues (Slurring /using the wrong word)
- Shortness of Breath
- Facial Numbness
- Facial Drooping (eyelid, lower lip)
- Right sided weakness
- Right sided numbness
- Tremors in the Right Hand
- Symptoms my mother thought was a stroke
- Loss of feeling from my lip to my mid chest
- Heat Intolerance
- Right Orbital Cellulitis (Behind my right eye)
- "Seizure-like" episodes

When the symptoms first began, my doctor assured me it was just stress and wanted to put me on antidepressants. After all I was a single mom and worked too much. I must be burnt out. Then I was diagnosed with a B12 deficiency and put on B12, but still my symptoms got worse.

I had my first major attack in January of 2010. When I got my first "attack" my face drooped on the right side (It felt like someone was pulling it down by my neck which choked me),

I couldn't open my right eye, I got tremors in my right hand, right sided weakness/numbness, my head began to "burn" (it felt like someone lit my brain on fire and closed the lid) which caused intense pain, and my muscles reacted involuntary. I forgot to pick up my feet even though my head thought I was, which caused me to fall and I misjudged distances and walked into things. Now, I also get palpitations (transient abnormal EKG's); my speech becomes slurred, and sometimes can't swallow.

In the early stages I was admitted to the hospital for massive antibiotic treatment and tons of labs. I had blood work for NMO, CBC, BMP, Celiac, a screening for Lupus (my ANA was positive titer 40 and speckled), and CT's (Negative), MRI's (Negative), EEG's (Abnormal x 2), and Spinal Taps (Negative). The doctors also noticed that my electrolyte levels go crazy and that potassium and calcium seem to be affected no matter what. During this time I also had my thyroid removed because of its size. I have had Hashimoto's thyroiditis since 2002, that was hard to control. When the surgeon got in there the antibodies had destroyed or "melted" the thyroid and it had to be dissected out of my throat....which landed me in the ICU.

Afterwards, I was placed on steroids for the swelling and all of my symptoms disappeared. Two weeks later they removed the steroids and all of my symptoms returned. I was referred to a neurologist after multiple progressive episodes, and he found that my antibody level was 2187. I had an abnormal EEG that showed left temporal lobe involvement, and it was clear that the steroids seemed to make my symptoms stop. It was then determined that I had Hashimoto's Encephalopathy.

After my discharge, I was placed on 4 mg of methyl prednisone and remained stable for 3 months but had residual function issues. Then, I had another episode which required 3 days of 125 mg of Solumedrol, 6 days of 250mg of Solumedrol, and a maintenance dose of 8 mg of Methyl prednisone a day. It is also around this time that I had bouts of an irregular heart rate. I have had abnormal EKG's in the past during Hashimoto's exacerbations which feel like being kicked in the chest and then it takes 3-5 seconds for my heart to "reset". I also have issues walking up stairs or with physical activity and with temperature regulations. They have attributed this to Postural Orthostatic Tachycardia Syndrome and also potassium/magnesium deficiencies.

After an episode/attack, I receive steroids and the attack usually stops. I often need 3-5 days of IV steroids for them to go back in remission. Steroids don't seem to stop them all together though because I have had 18-required issues in two years.

Over the past two years I have dealt with residual function issues of fatigue, tremors, dizziness, vertigo, head pain, unstable levels, muscle contractions, etc. It got to the point where I called my family at least 3-4 times a week because I couldn't get myself home. Stress, sun, illness, repetitive muscle movements, and activity made the symptoms worse. Then I started experiencing involuntary throat muscle contractions that feel like I'm being hanged and requires lying down to make them stop.

Here are a few before/after snapshots of my daily life and the effect Hashimoto's Encephalopathy has on it:

Daily Impact:

Before: I used to take driving and flying trips with just my son and me. We went to places as far away as Jamaica and England.

After: I rarely go anywhere by myself and when I do it is short distances for a quick errand. I do not like to drive long distances because it causes my hands and arms to go numb. Now when I travel, it takes a lot of planning and preparation to make sure I can get medical care, that I won't get overheated, and that I am able to stop frequently. I am also unable to travel for my job anymore.

Before: I used to go out with friends, do public speaking, and was very social.

After: I often times will skip activities with friends because of fatigue, pain, or the fear that my symptoms will happen while out. I hate that people have to leave places in the middle of things because I get ill or become overwhelmed with too much activity or stimulation like noise, sounds, and smells. Also, just getting ready can wear me out at times and now takes 2 times as long to complete. I no longer do public speaking because of mixing up words or forgetting what I'm talking about and then I get very frustrated. I also have issues with anxiety every day.

Before: I used to play sports with the kids at my job, go to the beach, and was always on the go.

After: I find it difficult to get up a flight of stairs or do physical activity without getting winded, palpitations, and my heart feeling as if it is going to beat out of my chest. I cannot stand for more than 15-20 minutes or my legs and feet turn purple and start to hurt. I can no longer enjoy outdoor activities because the sun causes blistering, overheating, and fatigue. A simple day at the beach or boating with my family now requires a "good" day, 80+ sunblock, ice packs, tarps, increased steroids, and then I can only be in the direct sun 15-20 minutes at a time if the temperature is above 80 degrees. Even simple stretching exercises can be painful sometimes. I have balance issues and often feel like the world is tilted on its side or moving.

Before: I used to work 60-80 hours a week without a thought to it and I was the go to girl for the organizations problems. I played sports with the kids and did all the administrative work for the organization. I lifted equipment, walked, ran, jumped, sit, crawled, and was always on the go. I ran trainings, did public speaking, and planned large events.

After: Over the past two years I had to take multiple extended leave of absences and have had to call out or leave work on many occasions due to medical treatment, hospitalizations, or symptoms. I started shying away from being on sites because of my immune system being compromised and the childhood illness exposure. I would go to work every day with some level of pain and would try to hold up which resulted in me holding my head in pain by the end of the day and 3-4 times a week having to call someone to pick me up or having to leave work to go lie down. Something as simple as use of my hands for typing, filing, or counting money caused tremors, muscle fatigue, and contractures in my arms and hands. Job stress whether mental or physical brings on headaches, fatigue, neuropathy (numbness), muscle pain, and/or tremors. I became unreliable due to the unpredictability of my health. Even when my head gives me a break, I have recurrent UTI's, kidney pain, palpitations, neuropathy, and blood sugar issues. I noticed that the more I do the worse things are. I often tried to hide symptoms from co-workers by sitting on my hands or down playing pain but they could always tell because of my speech and inability to keep going.

A typical day before I got sick: I would get up at 4:30am, get my son dressed, and go run a morning program for work. I would work in and outside all day playing sports with the kids, running meetings, and being an administrator until around 8pm. Usually we would go get dinner with friends. I would then take my son home, play, and then get ready for bed. I would often stay up until 11 pm cleaning, watching TV, or working. On my day off, I would take my son to the beach for hours and play in the sand. Then we would go to dinner and see a movie just the two of us. I also took him on frequent road trips all over the place. I never gave a second thought to not being able to do things, and every Sunday we would have big dinners for people who lived in my apartment complex.

A typical day when I was employed after getting sick: I would get up at 6:00 am to be at work by nine. I would often realize that my hands were not cooperating so it would take a lot longer to get ready and that, coupled with having to take medication spaced out, adds a couple of hours to the time I need to get ready. I am no longer able to wear "bands" without losing feeling in that body part. For example, my watch (hand goes numb), socks or heels (feet go numb), bra (chest goes numb), and stretch jeans (loss of feeling in my legs and groin).

By 9:00 am I might be in a meeting and feel tired from not sleeping well the night before. This means I have trouble concentrating and my hands begin to shake. I sit on my hands and begin presenting my information when I realize I sound "off." I take an extra 2 mg of a steroid to combat it but in the meantime I start having trouble swallowing and my face is drooping on the right side. Once the steroid kicks in I feel like I am sped up and I have begun to noticeably sweat. I am forgetting things and don't feel very well but at least I'm functional. By 10:30 am I may notice my blood sugar is low and I realize need to get something to eat because I am going to pass out. (This happens frequently.) By noon I need to sneak out to go lie down for an hour during my lunch break because I know I am not going to make the rest of the day. My back may started to hurt from the calcium I am passing in my urine, causing me to believe I am getting another uti. I might then try to get up and return to work but my head may be killing me so I call my boss to tell him I'm going to need to rest. He may respond that he needs me to do one site visit today instead, so I get up and drive out to a site. While I'm there things are getting worse and I have lost feeling in my chest and groin, and I feel really awful. Afraid that I won't be able to control my bladder, I call my fiancé (now husband) and ask him to please come and get me. Once home I lie down and the symptoms start to ease up. I get up and try to finish the work that I missed and am now too tired to cook. My fiancé offers to go out to dinner instead. While at the restaurant, the noise gets to me and we have to leave in the middle of dinner. Once home I am finally able to take Ativan which puts me to sleep. If my symptoms fail to improve, I often end up at the hospital, IV outpatient, or the Dr.'s office for treatment.

After two years of this roller coaster ride and trying to do it all, I realized that I was unable to work. On average 4-5 times in a five day work week my symptoms would warrant the need for me to be at home resting. I became unreliable and couldn't guarantee that I could be at a job during any certain time period. I have had 18+ hospital episodes in two years and that is just for the times I couldn't manage at home.

One day it might be kidney pain, stones, or a uti. The next day it would be GI complications from antibiotics or steroids. Then because of the stress, my symptoms would get severe and I would be fighting pain, tremors, neuropathy (hands, feet, chest, groin), headaches, blurred vision, slurring speech at unpredictable times because of fatigue, side effects of meds.

I would try to push myself to work a full week because of fear of getting fired and I would suffer because of it. The stress of trying to get places and appear normal everyday would lead to severe anxiety and unmanageable fatigue or pain, which meant I would have to call someone to come and get me because it felt like I might pass out or that my body would "shut off". Not to mention the stress of trying to keep up with 4-6 appointments a month with no time to take off.

When I would be forced to stay home because of the severe pain or issues I would try to work from home because I was scared that I would be fired or demoted. This resulted in not being able to rest and the symptoms would progress.

I still try very hard to get up every day and look presentable. It just takes me a lot longer. I have been fiercely independent all my life and it is a huge change that I am scared to go more than a few miles by myself because my symptoms are unpredictable. Two years ago I worked almost seventy hours a week and never stopped moving and it is very frustrating to now feel like I have the stamina of an elderly person. I have a certain number of things I can get done in a day then I'm out of energy and ability to do anymore. Sometimes I try to push myself to do something because I really want to be there for my family and I end up paying for it the next day.

I shy away from going out with friends because it is embarrassing if we have to leave in the middle of something because I am worn out or because I can't physically do what people my age can do like go to the beach, play sports, etc., all of which were my favorite things to do.

I was always a very social person but this illness can be isolating. It has also caused strain and stress on my family because of the frustration of having to depend on them to do tasks that I always did and the financial aspect of not being able to work. It is hard for someone who doesn't live with this disease to understand. My now husband is a huge support to me but it is hard to push away that feeling that I am robbing him of a normal life. He just laughs and says, "Why would I want normal when I can have you?"

One of the things that counts against me is because I am "young" and "pretty" (as I have been told) people assume that I must have perfect health but that couldn't be farther from the truth. I had to quit a job where I helped thousands of children and was the primary bread winner for my house because I knew if I didn't that this disease would take my life. My levels were all over the place, the pain with exertion was too much, and each of the episodes was more severe and incapacitating the more I try to do.

Since quitting my job, I applied for and was granted disability. I am now able to focus on my health, getting better, rest, and concentrate on the multiple appointments I have each week. I also realized there is so much more to me that just my job and that my life is far from over.

I recently got married to an amazing man who supports and loves me regardless of my limitations. As far as treatments go, I have traveled to Mayo and saw a number of specialists that recommended a lot of different things, all of which seem to fix something but break something else.

The thing I finally realized is with this illness doctors most of the time are flying as blind as we the patients are. Steroids help but de-stressing is better. A lot of the other therapies are toxic to the body and so I discovered that supplements, the thyroidectomy, and taking care of myself seem to be better avenues for me.

I still use steroids for relapses but I no longer take them daily. I am also trying an Immunocalming diet as well as treatment for candida. My antibodies have fallen to less than 100 which I believe is a major contributor to my improvement but I have no medical basis as to why.

I have a great team of "ologists" that are working with my whole body to balance levels and so far I have seen a major improvement in my quality of life. With HE it is easy to get caught up in the what if's and the need for guarantees, especially when you relapse. I can't tell you how many times I fear not being here, of not being able to regain myself after an episode, but then I realize I have no more of an expiration date than anyone else on earth. I am just more aware of mine. I refuse to be anything other than optimistic and believe that a cure is on the horizon as we start to understand more about why autoimmune diseases occur.

My biggest lesson is to be your own advocate and do your research. WHY's are important to me and my doctors as well. I can accept I'm sick but I want to know why. I came up with a few of my own ideas including a high stress life, the CMV and Epstein virus exposures, and the fact that I had received the 2009 double flu shot six weeks before my symptoms started. I can't know for sure but it is some of the things I have seen that relate to a number of other patients. I also have surrounded myself with outside-the-box doctors. I am the first one to tell the doctors that I am not the protocol patient, I didn't read the text books, and textbooks don't work for me. I need them to see me, the person…and not just HE

Gitte

I live in Denmark and this is my story.

In September 2009 I was in Norway for a month with my husband who was on job up there. During this time I felt tired - more than normal - and I decided to go for a check up at my doctor's when I came home.

And so I did. That day my ordinary doctor had a day off and his partner took the session with me. I had that day trouble speaking but wasn't aware of it myself. The partner who didn't know me thought I was a bit crazy and funny. At the evening I got worse and I was throwing up and my ability to speak got worse. We went to the Emergency and entering that I went into a coma-like condition and cramps. I have almost no memory of the next four days. The investigation by doctors was for almost anything: HIV; Creutzfeldt Jacobs - you name it.

But an intern had read something about HE and ordered a sample check for thyroid antibodies and it showed 75000. I got a spinal tap which showed irregularities.

They started me on 200 mg prednisone (oral) and I cleared up during the next two days. During the next month I tapered down to 50 mg.

The next year and a half I took prednisone at different doses. I get my bloodwork done every week and we regulate the steroids after the antibodies.

For a half year ago I got a combination of sadimun and prednisone because of the side effects and it helped a lot at first. But at the moment my antibodies have gone up again so my dose has gone up too.

Now the plan is to exam if IVIG is a possibility. We considered removing my thyroid but the results of that kind of treatment is not yet clear. I would do it if it would do the trick, but it's not clear so I have refused at the moment.

I have found that it's important to take calcium and Vitamin D every day - 2x 500 mg. Otherwise one's bones can get into trouble.

I take one tablet every morning to drain the water in my body - if you do so remember to check your calcium level every three months.

It's important, I think, to live as if you have diabetes in term of eating. Low calorie diet with a lot of fruit, fish and vegetables helps to keep the blood sugar stabile.

I use a lot of oil to keep the skin smooth - steroids dry it out.

There is an island woman who makes a very good skin cream (SOLEY). She makes it herself after a very old recipe from her country. I find it is good on the face where the steroids change the skin and gives us cheeks like a hamster.

The only way I have found to keep some form of track of HE is to get my blood tested. During these two years I have found that when my antibodies rise I can feel it. When they go above 6000-9000 my muscles and my head freeze in a way. A benefit to get the blood tested is to keep track of the side effects of steroids and sandimun also.

Once a year I get my bones scanned to check if the steroids have made any trouble - so far so good. I had my head scanned a year after to see if there was any track of the encephalopathy but it all seemed normal.

I take 200 micrograms of selenium every day. Research has shown it can have a positive effect on antibodies. I also take 30 mg beta blocker a day to keep my heart steady and my pulse normal. I take two lanzoprasol a day to keep my stomach happy. (Steroids can be hard on the stomach). And I take my ordinary meds for the thyroid.

I have decided to go without antidepressives and sleeping meds because I feel I dare not take anything that may affect my brain. That's my personal choice.

Sharon

I was born in Jonesboro, Arkansas, and my health problems started during childhood. When I was 6 years old I got the measles and my temperature rose to 106 degrees. I was in a coma for two days. When I came out of the coma, everyone thought that things would be fine.

One Saturday morning when I had been home about 4 days I was watching the Lone Ranger; and the next thing I remember was my dad looking over me and telling my mom to get my things because we were going to the hospital. On arrival at the hospital, they transferred me to LaBonner Children's Hospital, where after 5 days I was diagnosed with Epilepsy. I was placed on medicine and had seizures until the age of about 16, at which time the seizures stopped.

I finished high school and took courses in the Hospitality Industry, and I worked in that industry for 12 years. I was the first female General Manager of a hotel in downtown Little Rock, AR. When our Governor, Bill Clinton decided to run for

President, Al Gore took over 3 floors of my hotel and I got to meet a lot of celebrities.

At the age of 26, I became pregnant with my third child and was told to have an abortion because of all the medicine I was on. I did not believe in abortion, so I decided to have my child. My seizures had returned with a vengeance about 3 years earlier, and I was not in good health. However, I found a doctor that would take me on and I have a wonderful grown son now. He is the light of my life.

In 1999, I formed the first Epilepsy Education Association for the State of Arkansas. I was chosen by the National Epilepsy Association as the person that had make the most difference in that year, and they decided to come up with a new award: the "Making a Difference" Award. I was the first recipient. I have spoken before Congress about Epilepsy Education on two different occasions. I have been sent to Chicago and sent several other places to speak concerning Epilepsy Education. I was also given awards such as: Top 4 Women in Arkansas, Woman of the Year, and Arkansas Children's Hospital Award. I had also written 2 children's coloring books for kids at Children's Hospital.

All of this time, I had not been feeling well and had noticed problems with my walk, headaches and memory. In 1997, my PCP ordered an MRI and he saw an abnormality in the white matter in my brain and told me that I had MS. I was told I was doing well and that they would watch me, but I did have MS. I was told to get plenty of rest and stay away from stress. But over time one doctor would say I had MS and then another would say, well, maybe....No, you are doing too well.

I have also gone to school for Court Reporting, and I was a Court Reporter for 7 years. I also sold real estate for 5 years. I was and still am a motivational speaker, and I teach singing and playing the piano and guitar. Unfortunately, during the last few years, it has become more difficult to do these things and sometimes I forget the words of a song.

My health history also includes trouble with my bowels. Since about 1996, I had noticed that I was having a lot of bowel movements and it got to where I could not eat anything during the day if I was going anywhere because it would go right though me. I tried to continue working and would not eat all day, but I became very malnourished and started losing hair. They sent me to a rectal doctor and he did some tests and told me that I was going to need a colostomy bag!!!! I was devastated.

In June 2010 my first colostomy bag was put in. I got a staph infection in the hospital and was placed in isolation. In February 2011 I had a hernia around my stoma and had to go back into the hospital and have the hernia removed and my colostomy redone. In August 2011 I had another hernia removed from around my stoma. All of these times, I noticed memory problems, muscle jerking, and muscle weakness.

After my colostomy, they sent me to a gastroenterologist and he put me on three different medicines but I was still going to the bathroom about 15-20 times a day. I had to quit working and stay home.

I was sent to the Cleveland Clinic in Ohio to see if they could help me with my stomach issues. While I was there they talked to me about MS, and told me that I had an autoimmune disease. While in Cleveland, I saw a neurologist who ordered some tests, including an MRI and scans down the spine. He said that he would look over the results and let me know. We returned to Arkansas.

About a week later, I received a call from the head of neurology in Cleveland and he said I had Hashimoto Encephalopathy. He wrote a letter about treatment and I tried to show it to some of my doctors in Arkansas but they did not know anything about it and said I was not going to get this disease. I finally found a doctor at UAMS. He was taking my history and we talked about my low white blood count, thyroid problems and of course he noticed that I had weakness and a difference in the gait of my walk. He ordered blood work and then called to tell me I had Hashimoto's Encephalopathy.

I was started on 100 mg of Prednisone one day, and that was repeated in 14 days. After a while they changed the dose to 80 mg every 10 days. At present I am receiving 80 mg every 9 days, and I have an appointment coming up soon.

I am a pastor's wife, so I am in front of the church a lot, singing, and leading the praise team. We are very involved in our community and this disease has really taken a toll on me. I had just started to have less bowel movements each day and was changing into a small bag and hoping some day to be able to irrigate, but now with the prednisone, all that I do most day is go to the bathroom. I try to keep going, but it is very hard when your bag is full and you have no way to empty it.

The other day I went to my primary care doctor and he stated that he knew nothing about HE so he could not help me. I had a bladder infection and he had me call my neurologist for a prescription. He could not understand that. I am just grateful that I found someone that knows about HE. Well, I should say, hopefully he does.

I was diagnosed in September of 2012, but I do suspect that all of the white matter lesions that they saw in my brain in 1997 could have been HE, but most doctors in Arkansas do not know anything about it. It is a very hard and depressing disease. I am so thankful for the Facebook community of HE patients, and for my faith in the Lord.

Odell (age at diagnosis: 45)

As told by Susan Foley

Odell was diagnosed in 2005 with Hashimoto's Thyroiditis and at the same time they found lumps on his Thyroid.

In January he had a needle biopsy of the Thyroid, and within three days after the biopsy he developed neurological symptoms, including bilateral facial paralysis. At its worst, he had to pinch his mouth closed to eat. He experienced extreme sensitivity to light and sound, double vision, blurred vision, and his sense of taste was altered. Other symptoms included fatigue, drooping eyelids, which became so severe on the right side that at times he could not see out of that eye. He also experienced facial tremors and jerks, dizziness, difficulty with selecting words, peeling lips, eyes so dry that he would have to tape them shut at night, or alternately, eyes that watered so badly it looked like he was crying all the time.

Odell eventually went to the ER one day thinking he was having a stroke. When he got there, the doctors examined him and told him he had Bell's Palsy. They sent him home, but he later received a phone call informing him that his needle biopsy had shown cancer. Unfortunately, he was so ill with neurological problems that the cancer could not be removed until he stabilized. He had to let the cancer grow in the meanwhile.

In July 2006 his thyroid was removed. Doctors found that the cancer was massive and extensive. In September he received radiation treatment.

His neurological symptoms improved for a while, but then he began having trouble using his muscles. When he would use one set of muscles a different set would tense up.

He was tested for everything they could think of, including Myasthenia Gravis and Lyme disease, but all results came back negative. (HE is a diagnosis of exclusion).

His doctor eventually told him that the most likely cause was Hashimoto's Encephalopathy, and explained it was a condition in which the immune system antibodies attack the brain.

Odell's symptoms were confusion, disorientation, tremors, concentration problems, attention span problems, difficulty retaining information, involuntary muscle jerks, fatigue, coordination difficulties, headaches, episodes of stroke-like deterioration, episodes of articulation difficulties, word finding difficulties, and problems with coordination of his arms, hands and fingers.

Odell had pulse steroid treatment of 1000 mg IV infusions for three days in a row. He quickly experienced improvement in his symptoms. He could finally move his lips and his eyes stayed open when he yawned.

Odell knew that HE was not curable, and that it was a relapsing and remitting condition, but he hoped the improvement he experienced after the IV steroid infusion would last for a while. But as it turned out he needed additional treatment, so by trial and error they developed a regimen of three IV steroid treatments, followed by one treatment four weeks later, then one more treatment four weeks after that, followed by waiting four weeks and restarting the treatments.

Although the treatments had reversed some of the problems and had slowed his deterioration, he continued getting worse and in time the treatments were no longer effective.

To add to this, Odell's neurologist had requested that his PCP manage his steroid treatment. His PCP, however, did not feel comfortable doing so. During April 2009 Odell was having relapses in between the steroid treatments, and felt he was slowly losing ground. He noticed that he was stuttering or slurring his speech, and that his right foot would turn out while walking.

In November 2011, Odell's search for help went nationwide. He wrote letters to hospitals, clinics and other doctors. He continued to relapse and remit, and at one point he went to Mayo Clinic where they confirmed his diagnosis of Autoimmune Encephalopathy. The doctor there recommended IVIG in May of 2011.

Today Odell is still fighting his battle with cancer, but he feels the neurological side of his health picture is the worst as it presents a daily battle.

As of the date of this writing Odell is still receiving IVIG (Intravenous Immunoglobulin) every 4 weeks, which takes over 5 hours to infuse. Afterward, it takes him 3-5 days to recover.

For the past six months he has also been on Cellcept (Myochenlate Mofetil) which is an anti-rejection immune suppressant medication.

He frequently requires a cane to walk, and his tinnitus and speech are getting worse. He has problems with slurring of words, word finding difficulties, and stuttering. He is having increased seizure activity, facial twitches, myoclonic jerking, and shaking of his arms and hands.

He also has brain fog and breathing difficulties, and problems with drinking liquids. He has joint pain, motor control problems, and vision changes. He has very little energy left.

Odell has his own theory on autoimmune disease. He feels that autoimmune diseases could be caused from too much stress in one's life, as he himself has experienced. /

CJ (age at diagnosis: 57)

As told by Susan Foley

C J's journey is long as most Hashimoto's Encephalopathy stories are.

In the early 1990's she was diagnosed with scoliosis and spinal spondylosis, and at the same time she began to have gastric ulcers. Shortly thereafter, C J was also diagnosed with fibromyalgia by her primary care physician and her rheumatologist.

Between the late 1990's and 2000, C J began to experience extreme fatigue and increasingly serious muscle and joint pain. A scan showed 6 cervical disc compressions and 3 bulged discs which gave her a diagnosis of DDD with spinal stenosis. As C J puts it "my fatigue and pain level went to the point where it felt like my plug had been pulled and the backup battery just died.

It was horrible." She was also told she had CFE. At this point, as her memory loss and cognitive problems increased, she had a series of brain scans.

At about the same time, C J began to get rashes on her legs and the trunk of her body. Her face would get pink and puffy, as did her hands and feet. Her nasal passages and her mouth developed sores and ulcers. Her glands would repeatedly swell, and then go down again. She experienced randomly occurring low grade fevers. She would be constipated one week and have diarrhea the next, never knowing what to expect from her body.

C J's doctors ran blood panels, ultra sounds, CT scans, MRI's, MRA's EKG's, EEG's EMG's, Neuro/Psych Testing, etc. She was diagnosed with what they thought was lupus after a punch biopsy.

Her physicians could not figure out what was wrong with her, yet they all agreed she was sick. With mild cognitive impairment, primarily short term memory issues and partial complex seizures, they could not put all the puzzle pieces together.

C J became anxious, and in the fall of 2012 she decided to go to a teaching hospital where the doctors started all over with blood workups and MRI/MRA's. C J had more EEG's and her blood work showed that her peroxidase antibodies were at almost 700 and her anti-thyroglobulin antibodies were very, very high. The diagnosis was changed to mixed connective tissue disease, vasculitis, Hashimoto's Thyroiditis and Raynaud's.

Meanwhile, C J was having very worrisome experiences. One day when she was driving home from a friend's house that was only 5 miles from her own home, somehow she ended up on a restricted road of an international airport. The worst of it was that she was driving a well-known route home – minus the turn-off to the airport's restricted property! Normally, the property would have a closed and locked barricade. But this time it was apparently not locked, and she found herself driving down a twisty dirt road with no guide rails, which eventually would have led her onto the runways. At some point she jolted back to reality, and within seconds realized where she was. She had no idea how she got there. Her mind was blank and she wondered how she got through the gates without scratching up the jeep. Luckily, she regained her clarity of mind before she wound up on the runway of the airport.

For a long time C J was too afraid to tell the doctors about situations like her airport driving experience because she was afraid they would say she was mentally ill, and she would end up in an institution. But when she finally told her neurologist, he said she more than likely suffered from a partial complex seizure or global amnesia.

In the spring of 2013 C J received her diagnosis of Hashimoto's Encephalopathy. Finally the pieces of the puzzle all fit. She has been left with brain atrophy and significant gray matter loss (more than white matter loss), much more than she should at her age. There are also lesions and divots with signs of compression from old trauma (auto accident).

C J feels like many others who are diagnosed with HE: that she had it for a while before it was diagnosed. She has had autoimmune problems most of her life, especially after a serious car accident when she was in her twenties. These problems became progressively worse as the years went by.. Like so many HE patients, there was a time when she had so many symptoms it seemed as if people just did not believe her anymore because she "looked fine." And like so many, she knows that if the people who feel that way could have the opportunity to live just one day in her body, they would understand. She also believes, as do many others, that stress plays a huge role in autoimmune diseases. When she is under extra stress, her rashes break out, and her pain and swollen glands all come back in full force. But of course she knows life cannot be stress free.

When C J informed her primary care doctor that she had been diagnosed with Hashimoto's Encephalopathy, the doctor had never heard of HE and warned her against the only treatment options available for the disease.

C J recently began taking CellCept and prednisone for her HE Although she has been warned of the serious side effects, she explains, "I've made up my mind I have fight to this. I can't just let it keep attacking my body and not fight back."

Madison (age at diagnosis: 17)

The weeks leading up to April 22, 2013 had seemed a little off for me. I had upcoming tests in two of my classes, which would usually be my first priorities, but I had pushed that to the back burner. I was soon going to visit Boone with a few of my friends, so I blamed my lack of concentration on the excitement of that, although earlier I would never allow myself to get excited without completing what was necessary to make an A on the tests.

On Monday, April 22 I felt unusually odd. I remember sitting at the dining room table like any other night, doing homework with my supportive-beyond-words boyfriend when I called my mother into the room. I simply said something was not right and I then fell off the chair into her arms. She guided me to the floor and I was unable to move my body. After about 10 minutes I came out of it and was back to 'normal.' We decided we would see my family doctor if it happened again, but declared it as a fainting spell.

The next day I went to class, and my boyfriend picked me up to take me to lunch. I was especially frustrated this day because no matter how hard I tried to pay attention in class I found myself thinking of nothing. Some may say this is normal for a teenager, but for me this was off. We sat in the car and I stalled to go in to the restaurant because I felt as if I did not have the strength to get up. I felt my head drop, and was unable react to the blurs of action that was going on around me.

He drove me to my mother and we all went to the doctor together - I was unable to move my body. I saw the emotion of all of the people around me: the fear in my boyfriend's eyes, the helplessness in both my mother and father's, and the confusion in the nurses. This lasted for about 2 hours, and eventually I came out of it on the way to the hospital.

I then again felt normal. Countless blood tests, a CT scan, and an EEG later, we had no answer to this spell. The doctors sent me home and told me to make an appointment with a neurologist.

The next day I had another spell of paralysis at about midnight and again went to the ER, again with no luck. These spells lasted anywhere from an half an hour to an hour and a half and I would eventually come out of it and be seemingly normal again.

The next day I had another paralytic spell at about 2:30 PM and had an appointment scheduled for an MRI that night. It came back normal.

I had a neurologist appointment the next day. My grandmother had come in town for support on my mother's behalf, and she and my family were all sitting in a room at the neurologist's office. I again became paralyzed, and a nurse rushed to get the doctor. He gave me a shot of an anxiety medicine, and eventually I came out of this spell – unlike any other time. He sent me home with the anxiety medicine and told me to see a psychologist to discuss conversion disorder. I felt I couldn't take the anxiety medicine because of the way it made me feel.

By this point I had discovered that my neck had become swollen in a butterfly shape off and on throughout the day for minutes at a time. I had also begun to have muscle tremors of my shoulders and head so I went to my considerate family doctor, Andy, to discuss these things. He told me that this butterfly shape was my thyroid and that it was unlikely that I had conversion disorder, because I have never had a traumatic event happen in my life.

Conversion disorder, a psychological disorder which presents neurologic symptoms in physical ways, was looking promising to doctors who had not seen me grow up. But the idea was ruled out by my family and family doctor, not only because I had not experienced any traumatic events but also because I had now been given three different anxiety/stress medications and the only effect they had was to make me feel like I was taking pills recreationally. My family doctor wanted me to see an endocrinologist about my thyroid, but did not have an answer about anything else going on. He continued to brainstorm and called me in for repeated blood tests.

On May 15, I began to have a new symptom: my shoulders would jerk, which I was later told was myoclonus. My arms would also flail sometimes. I was prescribed Xanax to help with muscle spasms and that helped to some extent, but it made me feel bad.

On May 21, my head was violently jerking, and my neck continued to be red and splotchy and swollen. My mom began to drive me to the ER at Duke Hospital, which was two and a half hours away from my home, but the violent jerking stopped on the way there. I saw Dr. Grant, a neurosurgeon at Duke, the next day and he told me I was not in the right field with him. I needed to see a neurologist at Duke, but the wait list was extremely long.

On May 23 I experienced an episode that started with paralysis but then got crazy. I was repeating the same word over and over, my eyes darting back and forth. I had a strange "happy" look on my face, got very emotional, and had a child like voice and responses. I repeated words "no," and "brownie" many times. It was as if I were possessed like in a scary movie.

The next day I began repeating words again, had crazed big eyes, and muscle jerking. I began running through the house and doing forward rolls on the floor while holding my cat -crazy!

Day after day my symptoms were getting worse. It seemed as if I was taking an illegal drug, but my brain was making me act this way. Headaches were constant, and my episodes occurred again and again.

When I saw the endocrinologist, I was diagnosed with Hashimoto's Thyroiditis, a fairly common thyroid disease. I had the antibodies, and an over-active thyroid. The endocrinologist stated that while I have this disorder, it was not what was causing my odd arrangement of symptoms.

My mother proceeded to do her own research online. She came across Hashimoto's Encephalopathy. The description fit my symptoms and we thought, finally! Now we just had to get me diagnosed and treated!

If only it were that easy. Because HE is a diagnosis of exclusion, it can only be diagnosed by ruling out every other possible cause. This is unfortunately also the diagnosis for psychological disorders. Since this disease is so rare, many doctors I went to had never heard of it, and clearly didn't want to tackle a patient with this pending diagnosis.

After countless blood tests, two EEGs, an EKG, two spinal taps, two CT scans, and two MRIs, I still had no unusual test results other than my over-active thyroid.

Since everything suggested the possibility of Hashimoto's Encephalopathy, my family doctor consulted a neurologist and endocrinologist at Chapel Hill Hospital and they agreed to start me on a Prednisone treatment. I began with 20 mg 3 times daily. The first day I took this was the day before my high school graduation. I did not sleep the entire night before (because of the prednisone) and the next day fell asleep at 6 pm and slept through the entire night. I eventually tapered down from this dose over the course of a month. My symptoms never completely went away, and the side effects of the prednisone began to get confused with my actual symptoms.

Depression came in to play, I was very jittery and sometimes hyper, and very emotional. I also began to have extreme OCD-like behavior, which was very unlike me. The only trend that was noticed throughout the prednisone treatment was that the less prednisone I took the worse my symptoms got.

On June 24, 2013, after 3 days of severe depression, I had an unusual spell. I had gone to the bathroom and wet my hair, and my head began to shake violently again. I did not want to be touched and would not stop ripping up a piece of paper towel. It lasted for about an hour and afterward it was as if I snapped out of my depression spell in a matter of minutes. I felt better than I had in days and it was very weird to me.

The next few days I had several episodes of craziness lasting 1-2 hours. I hysterically laughed at things that were not funny: burning charcoal, thinking everyone I saw was Justin Bieber, wanting to drive with cows and horses on the road, etc.

I had looked further into Hashimoto's Encephalopathy on my own and read that it can cause a patient to go into a coma if left untreated. I became very frightened of this since I was no longer on prednisone and had many, many sleepless nights too worried to fall asleep because I feared that I would not wake up.

The days began to be very blurry. My episodes lasted longer and I knew that my brain was getting more foggy and worse.

I could no longer remember my friends, and I had no social skills. I could not participate in a conversation because I didn't know the things to say. Any time I was around people I took everything they said literally, and it took me several seconds to comprehend if they were joking or not. Nothing came automatically anymore.

My family doctor wanted me to be admitted to the local hospital since it was beginning to affect my memory and he did not want any permanent damage. I was so relieved when this day came. I felt like it had already gone too far. I was relieved someone was finally taking me seriously. This was hard for me to explain because I now had the thinking skills of a child. I could only focus on one thing at a time and I had to think about everything very hard for it to make sense. When I told the nurses I was confused I got very frustrated because they would ask me questions like "Do you know where you are?" "Who is our president?" "What is your name?" I knew the answers to all of these things but my higher level thinking skills were gone.

The doctors at my local hospital contacted doctors at UNC Chapel Hill and the UNC neurologist recommended IVIG because that is what they would do there. I began a 5 night IVIG treatment while at the hospital. After the first night I woke up with more color and my thinking was still foggy but seemed to be getting better. I still did not feel like myself. The next day also seemed to get better but I still had some head falling episodes and zoning out. The next day I woke up with the worst pulsing headache of my life and could not stand to have my eyes open. I was given synthetic morphine which gave me no relief but knocked me out. I woke up with the same horrible headache and was given Toradol through the IV and had instant relief! It eventually came back but was controllable with Toradol.

I eventually went home after my five day long infusion! I felt more like myself than I had in weeks but was still cautious. We were hopeful that this would be my only miracle treatment but were quickly proved wrong. My physically symptoms eventually came back after about a month and I met with Dr. Tennison, a neurologist at UNC Chapel Hill hospital. He decided to put me on a IVIG treatment every three weeks for a year. I have currently just finished treatment number 5 of these three week treatments. My symptoms seem to go away for about two and a half weeks and then physical symptoms come back until my next treatment. I recently met with Dr. Tennison again and he decided to start me on Cellcept as well as the IVIG, to hopefully fill the gap of the three week wait for the next IVIG. So far I have had no bad side effects from the IVIG or Cellcept.

Since day one of these symptoms I was forced to stop driving, going to school, working, and being a normal, independent teenager. I did not get to finish my senior year of high school with my peers, but luckily my teachers worked with me to help me graduate. I am still unable to drive until 6 months after my last symptom. This keeps me from working and has put me in all online classes, which is an option I'm fortunate to have. I was unable to leave for the college I had planned to attend, and am still living at home, dependent on my family and friends for everything.

This has been the most frustrating, intriguing, and difficult thing I have ever gone through. I have a new found respect for those who are paralyzed, for I understand the frustration that they face trying and wishing to simply be able to move and to be independent. I also have this respect for those with Tourette's who have muscle spasms, or spasms of any type which are uncontrollable. The embarrassment and the longing to function normally once again. This respect comes out most of all for those who are mentally ill.

In the spells I had which resembled a mental illness, I felt as if everything I was doing was normal, but I was still able to process emotions of those around me. I saw the ones I loved most scared of me. When I was in public during one of these spells, I got glares and strangers pointing at me. These looks caused me to stray away from all of my friends. I could not allow myself to scare them by seeing me this way. I abandoned the ones who love me most because of the fear that they may judge me the way that I was being judged by those around me.

Although this has put me through hell and back, it has taught me to never judge someone from their outside symptoms. As if the symptoms weren't difficult enough, all these people experiencing symptoms want is to be like those around them. It pains me to look back at the little things I used to complain about when there are people longing to be well enough to even have the opportunity to go to school or have friends who love them for who they are. This has been the greatest learning experience for me, and I now see everything in a different light.

Trish (age at diagnosis: 56)

As told by her husband

In 1987, Trish was diagnosed with hypothyroidism and began taking Synthroid. Two months later she broke out in hives, which continued for four years, but no one could identify the reason for them. Doctors at Mayo were puzzled, as were UW Wisconsin physicians.

In 2000, because of the hives of unknown etiology and her increasing sickness, Trish decided she would have to retire early from her state job. Before leaving, she needed to have a hysterectomy and to have her gall bladder removed due to complications in both.

Once she rolled out after the surgery absent her uterus and gallbladder, she had no more hives. She was symptom free and well. Her uterus showed eosinophil infiltration.

Because it was thought that the Synthroid caused the hives, she stopped taking Synthroid and did well until 2007, when she tested low and began taking Armour. This improved her TSH and she felt better.

In 2008, she started feeling bad again so she was back on Armour. She got worse, feeling very depressed and suicidal. We went back to see her doctor at UW Wisconsin and found her TSH was at 50. She began taking T3 and pulled out of the depression, and felt much better.

She then found a rheumatologist in Florida who started her on Plaquinel, stating that she had Lupus. It was discovered that while her TSH was now normal, her antithyroglobulin level was at 3500 and her TPO was at 430.

In 2009 she began to become very depressed again, was feeling suicidal, was hallucinating and losing a full day's memory. She began sleeping 35 out of 40 hours, along with hallucinations, and was having memory loss episodes approximately once a month. Sometimes she would be going down a road that was well known to her, and she would become lost.

After three serious episodes where she went into a coma-type sleep over a three month period, I (her husband) decided one Sunday morning that she was going to have to go to the emergency room. I called her doctor but got another doctor on call. I described what medications she was on and what her symptoms were. He said to administer steroids. I said she is not on any steroids. He replied that he would call in a 6-day pack, and said she should begin taking it as prescribed. Just 48 hours later she was symptom-free. I reasoned that steroids do not cure depression, let alone my wife's other symptoms. We returned to her regular rheumatologist, who said while her ANA was a speckled pattern, her ANA was just borderline and that he wanted to continue to treat as Lupus.

In 2010 I made an appointment at John Hopkins because she continued to relapse once a month, and she was taking the steroid 6-day pack each time. Neurologists at Johns Hopkins diagnosed her with Hashimoto's Encephalopathy. The endocrinologist switched her to Levoxyl brand name only. The endocrinologist said he had no idea why she was having the brain symptoms. She saw a rheumatologist at Johns Hopkins for severe pain in her joints, which had also been getting worse. That rheumatologist said to go home and swim in the pool, that her problem was osteoarthritis.

In 2011 she had ten trigger finger releases as her fingers were freezing up and some could not move and were very painful. No physician could find what caused the ten trigger fingers. I made an appointment at Mayo Clinic in Rochester with an autoimmune neurologist and rheumatologist because two of her fingers were still very painful and while the 6-day pack of prednisone was working to cure each episode once a month, she was suffering cognitive decline and persistent relapsing depression, as well as hallucinations.

At Mayo, the doctor said that her decline was happening because she was being treated only when an episode occurred. In between episodes, the cognitive decline was occurring. He said she needed to begin daily use of immune suppression. He said her PET scan showed hypometabolism, which indicated immune suppression. When asked why she had to have 10 trigger finger releases, the rheumatologist she saw at Mayo stated that doctors like to do surgery. The rheumatologist also said her problem was osteoarthritis. Then he investigated Hashimoto's Encephalopathy and stated, "so once a month, the pain sets in and you become goofy." We immediately fired that rheumatologist, writing the CEO of Mayo. Mayo demanded we return and see a different rheumatologist, so we saw another. We insisted on an MRI of the hand because he, too, said it was osteoarthritis.

The MRI results showed the presence of active synovitis. The autoimmune neurologist stated, "You have rheumatoid arthritis along with Hashimoto's Encephalopathy." But the rheumatologist refused to classify the joint and tissue problem, only saying it was inflammatory arthritis. Eventually we had to let that rheumatologist go and found another in Florida who said, "What else can it be but rheumatoid arthritis. There is active synovitis and we know she has an autoimmune disease. She had to transition off methotrexate as liver tests were extremely high. Then once off methotrexate, that doctor left her with no treatment for the Hashimoto's Encephalopathy. We let that doctor go when my wife had one of her most serious episodes and her nurse said there was nothing she could do.

It was at that same time Florida passed a new law regarding hydrocodone, a drug that was being used to control my wife's rheumatoid arthritis pain. The doctor was angry at the state of Florida said he would no longer prescribe any patient any pain medication, even though he knew rheumatoid arthritis patients were exempt under the law. He gave us two weeks to find another doctor to prescribe hydrocodone. When we questioned him, he fired Trish from his practice and immediately stopped all monitoring of all of her medications. He had been the prescribing doctor for all of her meds. The Mayo doctor had to step in and take over care. We then found a rheumatologist at Shands, University of Florida.

In 2012 the Shands doctor understood well what Trish has. He said Rituximab would likely work. Mayo wanted her transitioned off the prednisone to steroid sparing agents. The Mayo doctor said she should transition on to CellCept. She was maintained on a very small amount of methotrexate for rheumatoid arthritis until her liver tests went high again. Then while at our home in Virginia, the pain from her rheumatoid arthritis was so severe that we went to a pain doctor. That doctor put her on Cymbalta for the pain. While the Cymbalta did nothing for the pain, it brought her to 100% on the brain issues. While CellCept had her almost back mentally, Cymbalta put her 100% back, in combination with CellCept.

In October 2012 October, with Trish's autoimmune encephalopathy now under control, the rheumatologist focused on her rheumatoid arthritis. He said it was not being treated. He also said because the progression of her rheumatoid arthritis on the MRI looked slow, rather than switch to Rituximab, we would treat the pain with Hydrocodone. Both the Mayo neurologist and now the rheumatologist stated that Rituximab would be next for treatment. So we went to the family doctor who said we needed to create a base line for the inflammation and use Celebrex. He stated that it only makes sense to establish a good anti-inflammatory for what is an inflammatory disease. This way he said it might reduce the need for the narcotic. So that is where we are for now.

Trish did really well for over a year on the CellCept for the HE but it didn't do much for the Rheumatoid arthritis. Having both HE and Rheumatoid arthritis which immune-suppressant to use became a problem. After a year on CellCept for the HE she broke through with a worse episode. This time she not only had hallucinations and frequent on and off sleeping while eating a candy bar she was going in and out of consciousness. She would open her eyes and then close them. One time while the eyes were open I asked her why her hand and arm with the candy bar was shaking. She said it will not stop shaking and closed her eyes again. I called her neurologist at Mayo clinic and I got his nurse on the phone.

I explained her symptoms and said we needed some prednisone prescribed because that is the only thing I know of to fall back on. The nurse said to call her neurologist in Florida. I said there is none, that the Mayo neurologist is the only one, and the Florida doctor asked that us to call Mayo. The nurse stated she was not going to have the Neurologist contact us. I said OK, if not him, is there someone on call for him? She said yes, but I am not going to have him call either. She said we are open 5 days and are a clinic. Have her Florida doctor prescribe the prednisone. I said I had spoken with them and they said to call the neurologist, as he is the neurologist. She said in that case it will have to wait till Monday and the neurologist will call you. I said it is 5:00PM on Friday, are you saying to do nothing until Monday? She said yes, she is not going to hurt herself and someone will be there with her. I said yes it would be like someone in the 1960's on an LSD trip until Monday. I said I need to know from the doctor if it will be OK to do nothing and leave her in that state until Monday. She said she handles people with hallucinations all the time but she would relay that to the doctor and call back on Monday.

I then called the Florida Rheumatologist who prescribed medicines on behalf of the Mayo doctor and spoke with the internist. He then placed a call through to her Rheumatologist. The Rheumatologist explained what my wife had and said he was to prescribe a 6-day prednisone pack as that has always worked. Like in the past, once starting the 6-day pack she returned to her normal self in 3 days with no memory of any of the episode. Mayo called back on Monday and her Neurologist said through his nurse that he will issue her no further medication and she needs to see a physician right away in Florida. That until he receives a call from a doctor in Florida providing him with her status he will provide no more medication. I again asked if it was a good idea to do nothing in another such episode. They said they will let me know but never did.

Several weeks passed since the last episode and she saw her rheumatologist. The episode was explained to him and he said no, it is not a good idea to leave her in that state. That it could cause permanent damage and we will call in a prednisone pack so you always have one on hand.

Grace

I am a Doctor of Physical Therapy by profession. I began to seek medical assistance for my problems in the beginning of 2003. For over four and a half years I diligently sought medical assistance, going from doctor to doctor on their orders and my own personal research…from test to test…on drug to drug.

As the months and years passed, the symptoms continued to worsen, and answers eluded all. My function has declined extensively in all areas of life. Pain is mostly all I know. What I was experiencing were not headaches, not migraines, but rather something I call 'brain-pain.' This is difficult to explain. Because I have had migraines for years the doctors just persisted in telling me that I needed a different migraine medication, then, a larger dose. Then it was another, different migraine medication I needed.

Then, I was told it was all 'in my head' and I should see a psychologist. So I did, but even the psychologist could tell that something was clearly wrong physiologically – the doctors were missing something.

I went to another doctor…and another…until I found one that ran the tests that might lead them in a direction…any direction…and eventually the right direction.

"Just please help me," I pleaded. "I'm 'losing time'…blacking out…having hours of time that I do not remember at all… having total conversations, evenings with people that I do not remember, losing friends because they say things happened and I say 'I never said that' and they would respond with, "yes you did"…and they think I am lying to them…because I do not know what is happening to me…it is an unbelievable experience.

I have lost so many people from my life because they do not believe that it can happen. They say things like 'oh, how convenient for you.' Seriously, I would rather have a working brain actually.

I put myself through 14 years of college, and I will be paying those student loans off forever (they still will not even let me defer those – even with my illness - my brain and/or my doctor cannot seem to ever fill out those deferment forms correctly, and/or they do not acknowledge the disease because they have never heard of it.)

I have lost pieces of my past…pieces of my present that I can never retain for the future because of the way this disease affects my brain and how it processes long-term and short term memory makes relationships so complicated.

If you or someone in your life has not yet been touched by a neurological disease you will be some day, and you will be less stressed when it happens to you if you know how to communicate with that person and why they communicate the way they do.

I was sent from one doctor to another as they figuratively threw their hands up in the air and 'passed the buck' by passing me on to another doctor or simply telling me I was fine. Even when the very first doc, my PCP of many years, actually ran and received positive auto antibody tests and inflammatory tests he did nothing with the results. Now I can only ask why?

He told me he was going to call me with the name of a doctor he would refer me to, but he never did, even after I called him back and reminded him. He reiterated that he would call me back with a name and number but never did. Perhaps he didn't know what to make of my results... but he had also recently been promoted to covering part of a prominent aspect of a hospital and would be moving from his local little practice to the Medical Arts

Building next to this hospital, and was cutting his regular patient care time down from five days a week to approximately two.

So, as I found another doctor to try to help me, I did as I was continually told: I sought a psychiatrist, who told me there was nothing wrong with my mental state, and I should see an Internist. It was that MD who noticed something, as I sat on the end of the table while she wrote some notes. As she glanced up at me she asked "are you having trouble swallowing?" I told her I was. She asked if my throat was sore and I said yes again but, I thought, I've always gotten sick easily, it's just from that. She got up, felt my neck, walked out of the room, called a doctor and said "I'm sending her to you now, she needs an ultrasound and biopsy today.

That is how I found out about the tumor on my thyroid that turned out to be quite large. Then came all the blood tests. My thyroid antibodies were through the roof. Medications didn't seem to ever get right - still to this day - we have to pay super close attention. So many years later and out of the blue, my body just stopped responding to the thyroid replacement meds and the tumor/growth started growing again and releasing...something

I felt awful, worse than normal, but the endocrinologist didn't seem to hear me until I had gained 62 pounds in 4 months - I did not eat 62 pounds worth!

The first thing they insisted on doing were steroids over and over again, which unfortunately didn't work for me. This made many people not believe me, so I was left fighting my own fight the entire time. The neurologist told me the only drug she saw to show any promise in situations like mine, at that time, was IVIG. But you needed to do an entire peer-review of the literature to get it approved at least in part by any insurance and she said she didn't have the time to do it.

Well, good thing I went to school as long as I did and actually learned how to do that. So, that's just what I did and I submitted it to my insurance (back when I still had insurance). It was an awful fight but eventually I did get approval.

Then for my first infusion they had me go to a cancer center where patients are monitored and the staff know what they are doing. For the second infusion, my insurance insisted I had to have the infusion at home with a home health nurse, rather than at the cancer center. On the second day of that infusion they sent a different nurse who repeatedly complained aloud about how long my infusion was taking. I felt terrible and apologized, but what was I to do? When she returned the next day she decided on her own, without any orders from anyone, she doubled the rate of infusion so that she could get out of there faster. There were no orders for her to do this!

I awoke to find she was gone and I could barely talk, barely breathe, c not go to the bathroom (urinate after about 2 liters of fluid had been infused into me) and feeling the worst pain my brain had ever felt. I called my Nurse Case Manager who scheduled the delivery of my IVIG supplies - the only number

I could find – and she said, "Hang up, I'm calling 911, you are going to the hospital right now!"

In the hospital, it was discovered that I was in respiratory failure, kidney failure and I was diagnosed with aseptic meningitis. From then on, I learned exactly how my IVIG was to be prepared, I only had one specific nurse, and with my own medical background, I asked if with special training, I could be taught to do my own infusions and just have someone with me at each infusion just in case. I felt I just couldn't trust these people, and my doctors agreed to my request. Within a few months I had completed my training and was infusing myself.

That is, until, my COBRA ran out and they refused my appeal for an extension. Every insurance company I applied to denied me coverage, and there went my brain-saver.

This is not all of my story, but HE has taken my life, shaken it, thrown it, run it over, and removed many loved ones from it by a lack of education, understanding and empathy. The slowness of my brain for small, seemingly meaningless jobs is one of the most frustrating things about this entire HE experience. And the sense that out there somewhere is the real me...not this person who cannot do as she used to do, or as the world thinks I should do (because 'you look ok'). Illnesses that affect one's brain affect so much more than the regular lay person may imagine. I really am doing my best today and every day. I do hope this book can help others.

John

As told by Susan Foley

John has had a number of illnesses since childhood, and began experiencing migraines with auras when he was only 16. It was so bad that he sometimes felt he would die as he was seeing Zig Zagging lines in his vision. He began to experience more and more neurological symptoms, and in 1999 his nurse practitioner realized John needed more help than she could give him, so she referred him to a neurologist.

The neurologist sent John for many tests, which first revealed that John had high ANA antibodies and high DSDNA antibodies. At this point they diagnosed him with lupus, although this did not explain the whole picture because John had developed more neurological symptoms.

He was having trouble with dexterity, so they ran more blood tests and found he had phospholipid antibody syndrome. Now John started with even more frightening symptoms, including psychiatric problems.

John's symptoms seem to come and go over the next few years, which caused him even more problems. He would awaken with a weird feeling that he could draw a line down his entire body, a line that went from left to right. John was so unnerved by the strange sensations he was having that he went to his rheumatologist and told him that although he was only

36 he felt like he should be put into a nursing home. He was terrified.

In 2005 he was referred to the lupus clinic at Mayo, which marked the beginning of his HE journey.

John went through numerous tests as Mayo but they all kept coming back negative. He was feeling frustrated, just wanting answers, yet nothing was showing up. After a night of worrying about his negative test results he received a call from the head of the department of neurology at Mayo, Dr. Robert D. Brown. John pleaded with the doctor, explaining that they had to find out what was wrong, and the doctor decided to order a SPECT scan.

When the SPECT scan results came back they showed diffuse hypoperfusion in the brain. Doctors also found high TPO antibodies of 444. After all this time John finally had a diagnosis: Steroid Responsive Encephalopathy Associated with Thyroiditis, or SREAT. (This is the term used by some doctors for HE.)

John had never heard of SREAT but he was relieved to know he would now be treated. He started with 1000 mg of solumedrol (steroids via IV) which was given over a few days. He felt awful, was very depressed, and could not sleep. But the SPECT scan showed improvement within a month, which was great news for him after suffering for so many years.

John had a relapse a month later. He had a problem with his leg, which did not work or feel right. He was again given a five-day course of IV steroids at 1000 mg a day. Thereafter he received the treatment once every three weeks. He finally stopped the steroids and now only takes them when he has flares. He was also given CellCept, which he continues to take.

John says he still has flares now and then. His HE has never gone into complete remission.

III. Children and HE/SREAT

Some of the most heartbreaking HE stories involve children who develop the disorder. They often suffer seizures, which can turn deadly.

The following stories were submitted by parents of children with HE.

Meagan (age at diagnosis: 10)

Meagan was so full of life and like everyone else that has struggled with this terrible condition, it took us by complete surprise.

Meagan was a very bright, intelligent and active child. She was determined to be gifted by her elementary school during the summer between 2nd and 3rd grade, because of her consistent exceptional school work and National Testing scores.

She also was extremely active in sports including Gymnastics, Soccer, Softball and Tennis all of which she excelled and enjoyed.

In her 4th grade year, around March, she started having issues in Math... we later found out that it must have started after she took the Florida FCAT because her scores were in the high 4 out of 5 in both math and reading.

Her teacher said she seemed to zone out at her desk and was not remembering the basic computations of addition, etc. I noticed her having difficulties with homework and was upset thinking she did not want to do the homework but she was sure that was not the problem and she would try harder. I also noticed her hands trembling but I thought it was because she was nervous and thought she was in trouble.

On April 2, I was tired after work and laid down for a nap while she worked on her homework and her brother went down the street to build a treehouse. She partially woke me and said she was going with her brother to build the treehouse. I do not know how long but soon I received a phone call from my son saying that Meagan was ill and he thought she was dehydrated and for me to bring water.

When I got there, she was unable to walk, he carried her to the car and I drove straight to the ER. She was partially paralyzed but stayed conscious. At the ER, we were devastated, they are not used to treating children, thought she had a stroke, was not sure how to treat her and told me to call my clergy and family. Finally flew her by Bayflight to St. Joseph's Children's Hospital in Tampa.

When we got there, the ER doctor said he needed me to allow him to do what he needs to do and that he thought she had a brain embolism in her frontal lobe. They had intubated her and we had to wait. Later they checked again and said no embolism and a neurologist said she probably had a seizure and would wake up fine. She did, Thank God!!!!

So I was told she had to be on seizure meds and everything would be ok. We were so happy..... But within a month she had another seizure at school and was again transported to St. Joe's. They did a spinal puncture and found nothing wrong, changed her meds and sent her home after she woke up from what was now her second coma. The med's were a lot and took their toll but we made it through the rest of the school year and summer but I could tell she was not quite right.

By September she had another seizure at home this time and again was in a coma for days, taken by ambulance to St. Joes, another spinal puncture and still no answers, I was told probably will never know.

She was deteriorating cognitively and personality-wise. She was unsteady on her feet and had terrible tremors in her hands. Nothing seemed to bother her though - she had an extreme regression and small child like presence. I prayed and prayed and prayed, and checked with her pediatrician who was not really familiar with her because she was not a sickly child, but in February of her 5th grade year (2010) the pediatrician ran thyroid tests that were off the charts and suggested we see an endocrinologist.

Within three days of being unable to get an endo for an emergency visit, I noticed Meagan had developed a goiter and I drove her to All Childrens Hospital in St. Petersburg Florida because I was getting the run around from her neurologist's office that would not involve themselves with the thyroid issue.

All Childrens found that the goiter had no nodules and put her on Synthroid and we went home. I knew in my heart at that time that all of this was related, even though none of the doctors felt it was. I prayed and prayed, others prayed, Churches prayed and God led me to sit at my computer and type in Thyroid and Seizures and AMAZINGLY THE BEVERLY SEMINARA ARTICLE ON HE came up and I read the whole thing. I knew God had given me the answer!!!!

But none of the doctors listened and Meagan deteriorated until a seizure in April 2010 that left her in a coma for 4 days, but this time I had her taken to All Childrens again and requested a change of doctors to their hospital. A whole team started working on her case, but they did not want to jump to conclusions that it was HE. They ran so many tests, sent blood work to Mayo Clinic in Rochester, Minnesota.

Meagan had been intubated at our local ER and they had aspirated her stomach contents into her lungs and gave her pneumonia causing an additional life threatening situation.

This time she woke up 4 days after and she was hallucinating. It was another three days before she was better and moved to regular room. When we were allowed to leave, they found the pic line had busted in her vein and had to do surgery to get it out.

Within 3 days out of the hospital, she was not eating and all of her issues were amplified including her eyes vibrating in her head, unable to walk unassisted, etc. I called the new neurologist's office and said I was bringing her back and demanded they treat her for HE. Within two days in the hospital they did the spinal puncture again and found she had unbelievable high antibodies in her fluid and it was HE.

They started her on IV steroids even though the endocrinologists were trying to tell me not to do this. They were at her bed trying to convince me not to continue when my lovely daughter woke up saying she was hungry!!!! Within 3 days, she was able to state her name, address and everything as if she was back to normal and they all were so surprised that doctors came from all over to check her out. They had previously thought she was mentally retarded even though I tried to say she is well above average when she was WELL!!!!!!!!

She had suffered so many atrocious nose bleeds, she had times when she could not speak a sentence that we could understand and now she was My Baby Girl Back to Normal!

The steroids were awful on her body but we were able to wean her off most of the hard line anti seizure meds and she was weaning down on oral prednisolone.

By October 2010, she had a partial seizure, but never lost consciousness and the neurologist decided to add IVIG monthly. She was doing well on the IVIG and the neurologist had weaned her down to almost no prednisolone when April 26, 2011 she called me from the school nurse's office and left a message that she was dizzy.

I went to the school and we had to search for her. She was wandering aimlessly and I took her home, made her lunch, and laid down on the couch. I woke up when I heard something odd and she was having a seizure. She was taken to the hospital and flown to All Childrens. She was not responding like they wanted her and the next day took her down for an MRI. When the nurse came in and said they had a problem, Meagan's eyes were not responding correctly

The final hours of our story are very difficult to write. Perhaps in a subsequent edition of this book I will tell the ending more completely. Our precious, beloved Meagan died the next day, April 27, 2011, at age 11.

Paige (age at diagnosis: 10)

As told by her mother

Looking back I can now see that our first symptoms for HE began at the end of my daughter's third grade year which would have been in April/May of 2011. During the end of the school year my daughter Paige, then age nine, began to have a dramatic personality change. She no longer wanted to go to school, refused to do work and was all around moody and at times mean to family members. Getting her to go to school or finish homework became a constant struggle during the last couple months of school. This was very uncharacteristic of her, as she had always loved school and was for the most part a "straight A" student.

As summer came I thought things would get better, but things continued to deteriorate so I began taking my daughter to see a counselor. Her personality change had been very sudden and intense, and she had also started head banging, or would hit herself when angry.

When meeting with her counselor my daughter talked about kids bullying her in school. This became our starting point for helping Paige. We worked on techniques for anger, and for interacting with classmates.

As school started, I went to talk to our school principal in order to let her know what was going on, and what could be done to start the year off right. She was labeled as Severely Emotionally Disturbed at this time.

When school resumed, Paige was at a point where outbursts and melt downs were a daily norm at home. She was largely able to hold it together in public, but home was a whole different battleground. Nothing we did seemed to help Paige on a long term basis.

As the school year progressed, Paige became even more set against school. She constantly complained about other students picking on her. I think things were mostly the same as they had always been at school, but Paige had lost her ability to handle school and the children's remarks. Paige has always been physically mature for her age and from a very young age students and adults commented on how developed she was.

With school going so badly and no one at the school addressing the issues, we moved her to a new school in October of 2011 when she was 10 years old. Things went well at the new school for a while, but at home Paige's behavior was still a struggle. Towards the end of the school year, the behavior issues we had been seeing at home began to spill over into school. She got along with no one at school, and had begun stealing from classmates. I remember telling her at times that if she would just try I was sure she could control her mood and what was coming out of her mouth. She would tell me, "Mom I try but I just can't control my brain. I know I shouldn't be like this but I just don't have control at times." She had also begun complaining of severe headaches on a daily basis. Both her teacher and I suspected she was just trying to get out of class.

In May she also became suicidal. At one point I got a call from her teacher because she scared some of her classmates by talking about wanting to hurt herself and wanting to die. A couple of weeks later my 10 year old daughter pulled a butcher knife out of the butcher block and held it to her stomach, stating she wanted to kill herself. She had also begun threatening me, telling me that she wanted to hit and kick me and hurt me. Obviously at this time we were still seeing her counselor, but things were not getting better and I felt as if my once smart happy-go-lucky child had slipped away from me.

Then on May 24, 2012, everything changed. My mom was over helping me at the house that day, getting ready for a garage sale. Paige spent the day one moment lying on the couch saying she didn't feel well and had a headache, and the next minute feeling fine. I got on her that day because she refused to help. But because I didn't want to fight I did not push for her to get up and help. About 3:55 in the afternoon my mom left to go home for the day. My husband came home from work around 4:00, and my son and two of his friends arrived about the same time.

We had a busy night planned, so Paige went to the kitchen to prepare a bottle for her bucket calf and my son was going to take her out to the farm to feed the calf and pigs while I got ready for a meeting.

At around 4:10 my husband started yelling at me from the kitchen. My first thought was, "what has Paige done now?" (my first thought whenever the household erupted), but when he yelled again there was panic in his voice and he started yelling at me to call 911 that something was wrong with Paige. I picked up the phone and started dialing while running to the kitchen. Paige was on the floor struggling to breath and was unresponsive. She was already turning blue around the mouth. While we waited for the ambulance she started having seizures.

The seizures continued at the hospital, and they started to run tests. One of the first things they did was run an MRI or a CT scan, I'm not sure which. They also started giving her medication for meningitis. This whole time she was in a state of constant seizing. We live in a small town in Western Kansas, and it was soon apparent that she would have to be taken to a larger hospital. The EagleMed from Garden City, a town thirty minutes away, was called in to flight watch her to Wichita, Kansas, approximately four hours away. Before she left they intubated her and also did a spinal tap. Due to weight restrictions, I was unable to ride with my daughter but my mom rode along in the plane with my daughter.

When my husband and I got to Wichita we sat down with the doctors. Paige was in stable but critical condition. They told us they were worried that Paige was having a stroke because her blood pressure was so high. I believe it was 170 over 150 when she got to the hospital. However, they were able to rule that out because an MRI showed there were no clots. Nevertheless they were having trouble keeping her blood pressure down and she was still having seizures, and was on a respirator. By this time she was on full life support.

The doctors explained that they were trying to slowly bring down her blood pressure and stop the seizures, and had started her on two anti-seizure meds. Eventually her blood pressure started to slowly come down but, the seizures were still occurring so they said they would try one more medication and if that did not work they would put her on a pentobarbital drip and heavily sedate her until the seizures stopped. When the third medication did not work they put her in a medically induced coma which stopped her seizures. During this time she developed a high fever and pneumonia. The pneumonia got so bad at one point they did not think she was going to make it.

After about three days they started waking Paige up. This was a slow process and unfortunately as she started to wake up the seizures returned. At this point they thought it might be Meningitis or the Herpes virus, but both came back negative. They then called in infectious disease doctors to take a look at her. None of the doctors seemed to have an answer for what was causing her seizures and high blood pressure. To make matters worse, Paige's kidneys had started to fail.

On Saturday, June 3, 2012, the doctor called us in for a family meeting. They still did not know what was causing the seizures and her kidneys were getting worse. He told us there were no pediatric kidney specialists in Wichita, and that the adult specialist would not take her case. He also told us that he had been consulting with a pediatric kidney specialist in Kansas City at Children's Mercy Hospital, and that if her kidneys did not start responding in a couple of days we might want to think about transferring her to Children's Mercy.

Luckily it did not take us long to decide that we would consent to the move if she needed it. Fifteen minutes later the doctor came back to tell us that the new labs on her kidneys were back and the doctors in Kansas City wanted her transferred immediately if we would consent.

So for the second time in nine days Paige was air lifted to a new hospital. At this time she was still on a ventilator and a respiratory therapist had to go on the flight, so no family member were able to go on the flight with her. After they loaded her up we went back to the Ronald McDonald house, packed our stuff, and headed to Children's Mercy in Kansas City, Missouri.

When we got to Children's Mercy in Kansas City, our hopes were raised because when we saw her in the PICU she was off the ventilator. We saw this as a great sign she was getting better. They had taken her off because as she was becoming more awake she was starting to fight the ventilator. We saw her for a little bit and then tests needed to be run so we were asked to go the waiting room. After a couple hours we were allowed to go back in and we were devastated to learn that she was back on the ventilator. This was a huge blow to us and we learned that during the MRI and other testing that she was again struggling to maintain an airway and the seizures were coming more frequently again.

By Monday her kidneys were doing much better but she was still on the ventilator and still seizing. At this point the doctors had no idea what was wrong and one of the neurologists told us that they were re-running the herpes test, as at this point they were pretty sure the previous test had been a false negative. He also told us to prepare ourselves because odds were not good for Paige's survival, much less recovery. At this point we knew from the MRI scans from Wichita compared to the ones in Kansas City that there had been at least minor brain damage, mostly to the part of the brain that controls emotions or personality. The doctors also told us that if Paige did survive, she would never be functioning at age level again and that we would have a significantly mentally handicapped child.

On Tuesday the doctors pulled us in for another family meeting, which meant me, my mom, and the doctors. My husband had gone back home to work since his leave was running out. At the meeting we were told that they still did not know what was going on, but their plan was to call back in an infectious disease physician, and also an endocrinologist. We were also told that if nothing was figured out by Thursday that they were going to start her on IVIG treatment.

That afternoon, the endocrinologist came and talked to us about what things they were looking for. They were called in because my daughter, who is age ten, had the body development of a thirteen year old. They told us they really did not expect to find anything but were going to run some blood test. About thirty minutes later the doctors came back in and told us we had to leave. Her labs had come back showing elevated thyroid antibodies in her blood. They needed to do another spinal tab (her fourth) plus they were going to start her immediately on IVIG treatment.

We later learned that they could not even test her spinal fluid at Children's Mercy, but they had to find a lab elsewhere that could test her for the Hashimoto's antibodies. Later that evening we were told that they were looking at the diagnosis of Hashimoto's Encephalopathy. Needless to say, we were happy to finally have a diagnosis because now we could start fighting it.

The doctors told us that steroids were the preferred treatment, but that they could not start her on steroids until infectious disease cleared her, and that is why they gave her the IVIG treatment. Finally on Thursday infectious disease cleared her and they started steroid treatment.

During this time we looked for any information we could on HE but did not find much. From what we did find though, we could tell the symptoms fit. The sudden mood swings and change in personality, headaches, weakness on the right side, and high blood pressure. The doctors also kept telling us how rare this was, and all Paige's nurses and care assistants were given information to read about HE.

Finally, about 48 hours after the first steroid treatments, the seizures stopped and stayed away. Paige was also able to get off the ventilator and stay off. During the days that followed, Paige improved but it was still a very stressful time. As Paige became more and more awake she had to be restrained because she would try pull out her pick line and feeding tube. She also started random talking and singing, and was constantly moving her legs.

When she talked it was all just random, and she seemed to have no idea of anything going on around her. She was also started on a Methadone drip due to the fact they said she was addicted to narcotic drugs they had given her, and was having withdrawal symptoms. As Paige became even more awake she started to have hallucinations and would scream for hours on end, usually believing that sting rays or chickens were attacking her.

By this time she had moved from the PICU to the rehabilitation floor but could not start rehab due to her combative nature. She knew her name and knew me and my mom by then, but she was having short term memory issues and if overstimulated she would become highly agitated.

They said she was suffering from ICU psychosis so they put her on a rotation of Seroquel and Ativan. She would get one every three hours. We became clock watchers during this time, waiting for the next dose that could calm her down as she was constantly moving and was agitated.

During this time one of her doctors asked my mom and me if we were ready to take Paige home and give her 24/7 care, and that if we weren't we might want to look for a home for her. Of course I was not ready to take her home like this because she was still hallucinating and combative and having to be restrained to the bed.

Finally it was determined that the Ativan was actually doing just the opposite of what it was supposed to, and was what was agitating her. Once that was stopped she began to come around and was able to start therapies and we could truly see how Paige was going to recover.

Paige had four therapies a day: physical therapy, occupational therapy, speech therapy and music therapy. No one really knew what to expect but Paige did wonderfully. It was like watching a baby make those first milestones, but in Paige's case she was making years of progress in days. She was only in a wheelchair for about three days before she was walking with a walker or just a gate belt. Before no time she was dressing herself, bathing herself and pretty much doing all her grooming herself. Mentally she was a little slower coming around and was having short term memory issues but overall progressing well.

Finally, after thirty-four days in the hospital, we were able to come home, with outpatient services for PT, OT and speech at home. She progressed quickly through PT and was done with it by the end of July. She finished with her speech, OT and counseling by late September into early October.

When she first came out of the hospital her medications consisted of Prednisone 80mg a day; two antiseizure meds, Keppra and Vimpat; and Amlodipine for high blood pressure. The Prednisone had many side effects. It left Paige unable to sleep, so a sleeping medication, Clonidine, was added to help her sleep. The steroids also caused massive weight gain of about 80 pounds total. Her Prednisone was on a taper, and she was supposed to be off in December of 2012. However when we got down to 20mg of Prednisone a day her symptoms started to return.

She started to have headaches and tremors in her hands returned. So her dosage was upped to 35mg a day and her taper slowed. She finally got off the steroids in February of 2013.

Since then no symptoms have returned, and she has started to lose some of the weight. We have just recently found out that the steroids have also affect Paige's bones and she now has osteoporosis. We go to the neurologist every three months, and also see an endocrinologist. We will go back in May of this year and are hoping to be able to take her off the sleeping medication and high blood pressure medication.

Her mood swings have also improved tremendously since getting off the steroids. For the first time in a long time we have laughter in our household again.

Before she could return to school we had an appointment in Wichita with a neurophysiologist to see what, if any, special needs Paige would need in school. Academically Paige was left pretty much unaffected by the brain damage but emotionally it had a huge impact. Paige was able to handle a day of school pretty well. The only adaptations we made were to her Physical Education, and to recess.

She could not participate in any activity that could cause a risk of a blow to the head so no volleyball, basketball or any other mildly contact sport in PE. She also did not go out to recess because of the heat. The steroids caused her to overheat very quickly and to turn bright red. The steroids also made her so hungry that she had to have a snack in the middle of the day to make it through school.

At home, however, she was very needy and needed a lot of reassurance and time. I had started my first year teaching but stepped down to be able to better meet Paige's needs at night. This was hard on the whole family but I had to do what was best for her, and my school district worked with me. I now have a different position within the district.

Paige has progressed so much over this school year emotionally and for the most part is back to her normal independent self - so much so that I am looking at getting back into the classroom.

This whole experience affected our family in many ways. While our family has always been spiritual, this has made us believe even more in the power of prayer and in miracles. I believe that so many people were praying for Paige that God listened and decided that her job on Earth was not done. Paige also made the decision when we returned home to get baptized in the church. She said that God spared her life and she wanted to show her thanks and praise to Him by being baptized.

This has also been a very humbling experience for us; so many people stepped up to help us in so many ways. One of the nice things about living in a small community is that when help is needed everyone steps up to help. Our whole community and surrounding communities all stepped up to help offering prayer, financial support and emotional support for our family. Paige received so many cards and gifts that they overflowed her room. When we left the hospital it took three carts to haul everything down out of her room. While in the hospital we got to meet one of the mail ladies at the hospital. She came to meet Paige because she said she had never processed so much mail before for one patient. The cards were a huge support to Paige and made her work harder to get home.

Paige today likes to pay forward what she received. Whenever we go back to the hospital for appointments Paige always likes to bring something for the staff or patients. This year she asked that we take a hundred dollars from our Christmas fund and spend it on toys and gifts for children in the hospital so we did. She had the biggest smile on her face when we took all the toys to the hospital after Thanksgiving.

We have also slowed down since getting home, enjoying more family time. I guess you can say that we now take time to smell the roses. We also appreciate more of the small things in life. I have also learned not to care so much about what people say or think. Many people have taken it upon themselves to comment on Paige's weight gain and puffiness. Our response to that is we don't care what you think, it's better than our alternative. Paige also regresses in maturity at times and almost always caries her favorite stuffed animal with her even though she is eleven. This would have bothered me in the past but now I really don't care. If she needs the stuffed animal to help her deal then fine, she can have it.

Paige is just finishing up her fifth grade school year and has done really well overall. The improvements over the year have been amazing. She continues to amaze me every day with her grace and optimistic attitude that she has shown throughout this recovery. She is looking forward to hospital free summer this year and the start of her sixth grade year, where she hopes to start participating in sports again.

One of my biggest frustrations once we got her diagnosis was the lack of information available to us. Most the time her doctors could not tell us what to expect, or her chances of recovery. The most common thing we heard from her doctors was, "We don't know. This is so rare that we just don't know."

I truly believe that Hashimoto Encephalopathy is not as rare as doctors think, but instead is frequently just misdiagnosed. I hope by sharing my daughter's story that I can help change this. If we did not get this diagnosis and started on the right treatment there in no telling where my daughter would be today. Probably she would either be dead or in a school for children with severe emotional problems.

Rose
As told by her mother

Our daughter, Rose, was a preschooler when we began to see the symptoms of what later turned out to be HE.

In 2007 we began to notice Rose suddenly falling and making no effort to stop her fall or brace herself. We referred to her as "limp noodle falls" because she would simply go limp and fall. She would also suddenly lose bladder control. She would appear to rather strangely "zone out" at times, sometimes in the midst of conversations. Although we took her to the doctor repeatedly, no cause was found for her symptoms. And so we began the long process of specialist referrals.

Four years later, on June 16, 2011, when Rose was seven years old, she lost consciousness while at school. It took two hours for her to regain the ability to talk, and even longer for her to be able to walk. She was admitted to the hospital for four days for the purpose of investigation, but no real answers came.

For months afterward she complained of daily, constant headaches, described to us that she felt as if the inside of her head was blurry, and he suffered varying levels of dizziness. Throughout the summer, Rose would continue to have sudden lapses in consciousness and/or abilities. For example, she would suddenly not remember how to read numbers, would wander off and not know how she got somewhere, repeatedly ask the same questions or tell the same stories. She lost the vision in right eye, and the right side of her face drooped for approximately eight hours on two different occasions.

Over time her symptoms became more pronounced, and began to occur with greater frequency. By this time, in addition to the symptoms I mentioned earlier, she was having sleep disturbances – waking multiple times throughout the night – and short term memory issues. Her emotions became extreme. She would experience sudden, overwhelming feelings of tiredness, intense cold, and weakness, as well as varying levels of ability to speak and walk. During these periods she would be extremely clingy, curl up on any flat surface and fall into a deep sleep that would last for three to four hours.

All of this took a toll on her school life. When these episodes occurred at school, she would be sent home. Some mornings she would wake up already headachy, overtired and sick feeling, and wouldn't even make it to school. Rose missed over 50% of her school year, and was experiencing chronic pain. She was unable to continue her training as a competitive gymnast because she could not keep up with the training schedule, and had balance issues which became more pronounced, causing safety concerns. She finally became so weak that she often ended up in a stroller or wagon by the end of the day.

In the course of investigation Rose had numerous tests, including MRIs, EEGs, VEEGs, ECGs, CT SCANs, heart monitoring, and many forms of bloodwork.

Almost five years after the symptoms began, and fifteen months after they became severely escalated, Rose was finally diagnosed with HE at the Mayo Clinic in Rochester, Minnesota by Dr. Suresh Kotagal.

We had struggled for almost 5 years trying to get first the pediatrician and then various specialists to take Rose's symptoms seriously; to acknowledge that there was something going on in her little body. Once her symptoms accelerated and began to change we became much more aggressive.

In Canada you must get a referral from your family doctor to see a specialist, and very rarely do you get to decide which doctor you are going to see. Getting an appointment with a specialist is notoriously difficult and involves a long wait. A pediatric specialist usually has at least a six month wait. At one point we were told it would be two years before Rose would be able to get an appointment to see a Pediatric Neurologist!

Each appointment would require more tests which took time to book and then more appointments to get the results and then more tests; only to be told that "yes, there is something going on with her, but we just don't know what it is." And then another referral to another specialist and another long wait.

Throughout all this waiting, Rose was continuing to have multiple episodes each week if not each day. Her symptoms were continuing to escalate and evolve. We never knew what was going to happen next. It felt as if we were always waiting for the next thing to go wrong and feared that we might be running out of time.

One day while in the middle of yet another marathon research session, I found the link to self refer to the Mayo Clinic. I was hesitant at first, but then figured we had nothing to lose. I sent the paperwork in not really expecting much of a response. I was very surprised to get a request to forward her records to them. Within a few short days, on May 25, 2012, we received confirmation of a week-long set of outpatient appointments to begin on August 7, 2012.

Of course, along with this good news came the realization that all of this would cost in excess of $15, 000 - money we did not have. So began a whirlwind three months of fundraising. Our friends, family and community came through in an amazing way and we raised enough to get Rose and me to Minnesota. We stayed at the Ronald McDonald House at night and spent our days at the hospital. We had one doctor overseeing her case and a variety of specialists that all reported back to her. Finally, they looked at Rose as a whole person not just individual symptoms! And within days we had her diagnosis.

Our naïve plan had been to travel to Mayo Clinic for the diagnosis and then return to Ontario for treatment. Never in our wildest dreams did we imagine that a diagnosis given by the world renowned Mayo Clinic would be discounted by the very doctors who had been unable to offer any diagnosis at all. We had thought a diagnosis from the Mayo Clinic would be the end of the struggle, when in fact, the struggle became even greater.

Where before the Mayo Clinic we were viewed as mildly over reactive, possibly pushy parents, now every word out of our mouths was met with derision and suspicion. Going out of country for a second opinion had made us persona non grata.

This despite a diagnosis from one of the world's greatest hospitals! Rose's MRIs showed atrophy in the right hippocampus, and white matter changes. Her EEG's and VEEGs were abnormal and showed "bilateral frontocentral temporal epileptiform discharges." Her blood work showed thyroid antibodies above 1,300, elevated TSH, elevated Anti-TgAb, elevated Esinophils, elevated IGE, elevated lactate dehydrogenase, a decreased white blood cell count, decreased RDW, and decreased neutrophils.

Despite all this, we are still fighting for treatment for Rose. Doctors in Canada have been unwilling to accept a diagnosis made in the USA. The Canadian doctors disbelieve the diagnosis and are only willing to treat Rose's Hashimoto's Thyroiditis and her epilepsy/seizure disorder.

Since August 2012, we have had to increase Rose's medications five times to try and "control" her symptoms. The doctors tell us this is within normal parameters and repeatedly state this will be the norm for her for the rest of her life: constantly increasing the dosage as her body grows and changes.

Today, Rose still has symptoms, which now also include hallucinations. School remains a struggle for Rose, in part because her high absenteeism makes staying up to date difficult. Rose requires a nap/rest period every day at school to be able to make it through the day. This means she misses out on playing outside with friends at lunchtime. She was unable to ride her bike for over a year due to daily severe dizziness.

She is under weight and has dropped down to the 10th percentile for her height. Most days she has little to no appetite, and receives supplementation to ensure adequate nutrition. Her friendships have deteriorated because other parents are unwilling to accept the perceived risk of having her over to their houses. Rose has little opportunity for independence because she needs supervision at all times. She has weekly and bi-weekly appointments to the Chiropractor and Massage Therapist to treat her chronic pain.

Sadly, every day presents some sort of problem, hardship or trial for her. What used to be easy is now hard. Schoolwork that she understood yesterday seems like new information today. Just getting out of bed is beyond her some days. Perhaps even worse, on days when she is feeling good and goes to school or to participate in a fun activity, she continues to have episodes that force her to have to walk away from it all yet again.

In some ways, Rose does not remember a time in her life when she did not feel like this; when the symptoms were not a part of her life.

In other ways, she feels it is not fair that all of this is happening to her and she has no control over her life.

She currently cannot participate in many recreational activities and she finds this very disheartening.

As a mother, I find this entire journey to be very emotional. I know and have known that there was something wrong with my daughter for many years. Yet despite repeatedly going to doctor after doctor, my fears and concerns were discounted. We as a family have had to fight, argue, research, educate and advocate for her every step of the way, and there is no end in sight. There are days that I weep tears of frustration as I must do battle yet again with an arrogant doctor. Other days I weep in sadness as I see that panicked look in her eye when she realizes she doesn't remember the last couple of hours. I feel like screaming and throwing temper tantrums when I have to meet with school officials yet again to advocate for her so that she can receive the basic help she needs, or a quiet dark space for her rest period. And I feel overwhelmed and dejected when I think of the struggles yet to come for her and us.

Rose's relationships with her siblings is at times negatively impacted as dealing with her issues, doctor's appointments, etc. takes up a lot of our time, and they feel overlooked or less important. Family outings and events are planned with her limitations in mind, and/or have to be cancelled, modified, or cut short based on how she feels. But in other ways it has strengthened the bond between them. They are all very protective of her and care for her deeply. Her many appointments and hospital admissions are made easier by their love and compassion.

Rose is fortunate to have a best friend, and that relationship has become even stronger through Rose's struggles. Her BFF is a constant source of encouragement and love. They are together a couple of times a week and have sleepovers at least twice a month. Her friend's parents have made every effort to learn as much as they can about Rose's diagnosis and have made her their honorary daughter. When they are together and Rose has an episode, they snuggle up in bed together and her BFF reads to her until she feels better, or they cuddle on the couch and watch movies until she regains her strength.

One of our greatest frustrations in all of this is the medical community's unwillingness to look at Rose as a whole person not just the individual symptoms. We feel she would have received a diagnosis and treatment much sooner if all of her symptoms were taken into account not just each specialist's focus.

Another frustration was the blinders the doctors wore to the idea of a rare disease. Just because it is rare doesn't mean she doesn't have it! Of course that is if a doctor even "believes" HE exists. Add to that, to diagnose a child with a rare disease that is under diagnosed in children! It is almost impossible!

Now, almost a year later, they continue treating only the symptoms, and we continue to search for a doctor who is willing to treat the root cause of her problems. While we search, her current doctors continue to waste valuable time arguing about the validity of her diagnosis, without offering up any other viable options. Are we upset and worried? Yes. And so we wait to see what will happen to our daughter next.

Julie (age at diagnosis: 14)

As told to Susan Foley by Julie's mother

Julie was 14 years old, in 6th grade, when things hit hard out of the blue.

Julie was in a severe car wreck in February of 2011 which caused her to need emergency gallbladder surgery. Just six months later she returned to the emergency room at the children's hospital in their town with strange symptoms which puzzled the doctors, who were unable to provide any answers.

She had developed a high fever and was acting strangely, exhibiting confusion, balance problems, and stroke-like symptoms. The physicians told Julie's parents it was probably just the flu, and that they should go home and if things got worse to bring her back in.

Her worried parents took her home, and Julie began vomiting. In addition, her other symptoms were getting progressively worse. In the back of Julie's parents' mind was the fear of meningitis, and they just hoped they were wrong.

Later that weekend, on Sunday, Julie's parents took her back into the ER, and by 11:30 p.m. doctors had ordered a spinal tap, which came back negative. The doctors admitted Julie to the hospital, not knowing what was going on.

On Monday morning a neurologist came to see Julie. He reviewed the blood work results and examined her. He looked at her medical history, which included Hashimoto's Thyroiditis as well as autism, ADHD clinical depression, mood disorder, OCD, Pandas, Hypogammaglobulimenia, PCOS and RSD.

He told Julie's parents that her TPO antibodies were "through the roof." That, along with her health history, led him to diagnose Julie with Hashimoto's Encephalitis. Julie's parents had never heard of HE, and worried what it meant. She had been on several different medications to treat her previously diagnosed disorders before this new diagnosis was added.

Julie spent five days in the hospital. Her MRI showed swelling of the left temporal lobe, and her EEG showed extreme slowing. This helped confirm the neurologist's diagnosis of HE.

When she was released to go home she continued taking high doses of prednisone, which caused her to gain 40 pounds. Julie is still getting IVIG Infusions every three weeks.

She is now 16 and has severe migraines, for which she takes medication. Her medication list consists of Synthroid, Zoloft, Clonidine, Topamax, 2000 i.u. of Vitamin D, Nortriptyline, Metformin, Spironolactone, Srattera, Gabapentin and Gamunex.

Julie's life requires her to see specialist after specialist, in a seemingly endless stream of appointments. She sees a neurologist once a month and has yearly MRIs and frequent EEGs, as she also has Absence Seizures. She was also recently diagnosed with polycystic ovarian syndrome.

Since the diagnosis of HE, Julie suffers severe daily headaches, and has become very slow in everything she does. She is still suffering from balance issues and experiences brain fog. She is also very forgetful. Her mom says that the diagnosis of HE has affected every aspect of Julie's life. Nevertheless she describes Julie as "a wonderful soul and a real trooper."

Because of all Julie has been through, including having multiple chronic illnesses at a young age, she sees a psychologist to help deal with depression. She is also now getting Biofeedback therapy, which her mother believes is having an amazing effect on her. She has also started a pain management regimen which is also helping. She is home-schooled by her very dedicated and loving mother who says, "I have not always been a strong person, but when it comes to your own loved ones who are sick, your child, you become strong."

Amber (age at diagnosis 17)

As told by her mother

On July 13, 2011, Amber and I were shopping for clothes and I said, "Okay let's go try this stuff on."

I turned to go to the dressing rooms and I heard Amber bump into a clothes rack and mumble something. When I turned back around she was falling down and having a grand mal seizure. She had never had a seizure before this. During her seizure she stopped breathing and turned bluer than a Smurf. I hope I never see that again.

I called for someone to help and thank God people did come to help. First responders came tried to help Amber, and all we could do was try and keep her from hurting herself further. Even though she stayed in a seizure the whole time, the people helping felt that Amber was responding to the sound of my voice, so I laid on the floor with her assisting anyway I could with the first responders until the ambulance came to help. It took the two first responders and the two ambulance crew to get her into the ambulance and get her stable enough to move to the hospital. Her breathing was so bad. It was like she was gasping for air the entire time.

At the hospital they had to secure her airway and intubate her. The doctors gave her medications to keep her in a coma so she should have been motionless, but despite that her body was still having tremors (shaking uncontrollably) or was still seizing. The doctors didn't know why this was happening.

She was life-flight to a bigger hospital (Toledo Children's Hospital, PICU). After what seemed like a billion tests for one and a half days, they decided to let her wake up from her coma. However, Amber was not waking up even after they stopped the medications that kept her out. The doctors had no idea why she wasn't waking up and told us they didn't know what condition (i.e. how much brain damage had been done) she would be in if she did wake up.

While she was in her coma I saw her lying there but I did not feel as if she was truly there in her body for a couple days. Then I started feeling she was there but not yet awake. (It is hard to really explain this). When I told the doctor this I felt like he must think I was crazy.

Then finally, (after what seemed like forever) a few days later the doctor got a response out of her. Her response was that she slapped him! I apologized for her and the doctor said that was okay because he wanted a reaction and he got one. He said she is a fighter. After she was extubated the doctor asked her why she wouldn't wake and she said she was tired and wanted to sleep and was mad at him for waking her up.

After all the testing, including spinal tap and drug test, all they found was that her thyroid was out of whack. They found she had the thyroid antibodies and she was diagnosed with Hashimoto's Thyroiditis. Because they couldn't find anything else causing her issues and was doing much better she was sent home with thyroid medicine and seizure medicine.

Amber seemed to be doing alright at first, but we were told not to leave her alone at all, not even for showering. We had to go back to work and thankfully her boyfriend helped and spent time with her when we had to work. He is such a blessing to us. On July 24, 2011, after I got home from work (Amber was with her boyfriend), she called me on the phone and was upset and slurring her speech. She told me she couldn't feel her legs. I asked her where her boyfriend was and she said, "I don't know." I then asked her where she was and she said "I don't know."

I knew she was in one of two places, and I asked her if she would be able to hang up from me and dial 911. She said "no." Anything I asked her the answer was either "I don't know" or "no". The next thing I knew we were disconnected. I tried calling her back. No answer. I got my husband and told him what was happening and we both got in our cars and started driving to the locations. I tried calling her boyfriend and my husband called 911, and learned that Amber had indeed dialed 911. An ambulance was in her area, but couldn't find her right away because she was on her cell phone and not a land line. The ambulance did eventually get to her and we met her at the hospital emergency room. This happened when Amber had awaked from taking a nap.

At the hospital the paramedics told me that they could not believe that Amber was able to dial a phone for help in condition she was in when they got to her. By the time she got to the ER she could feel her legs again. At the ER Amber's blood pressure was 96/39, that was a little scary. She had slurred speech so the hospital did drug tests (no drugs in her system other than the ones prescribed) and other blood work. She had an imaginary phone conversation. I had all the cell phones, but she told us all to be quiet because she was talking to so-and-so.

She was unable to scoot back in the bed (she said she didn't know how). She had to get out of the bed and walk around it and then sit back down where she wanted to on the bed. I thought the nurse was going to jump out of her skin when she saw Amber get up.

The doctors found out that the seizure medication was not absorbing into her system (at first they thought she wasn't taking it). She was put on a different seizure medication and transferred back to Toledo Children's Hospital that night. The next morning, July 25, 2011, all the doctors start coming again, and we were informed that they believed she has Hashimoto's Encephalopathy (HE). We said, "What's that?"

The neurologist explained it to us (of course we looked it up on the internet after he left) and said they would like to start Amber on intravenous immunoglobulin ("IVIG") treatments. He said it would be a 12 hour infusion each day for 4 - 5 days, depending on how she responded to the treatments. She only received 3 days of that treatment, as she responded very well. Her speech improved dramatically. Some of the other symptoms improved as well.

During this stay in the hospital my husband I went to the cafeteria to get something to eat and the nurse was with Amber, when we got back to her room about 30 minutes later we saw that she wasn't in bed. I instantly felt panicked, but upon entering the room we found her up against a wall not moving, she was just standing there. I asked her what she doing and she said she needed to go to the bathroom (which was on the other side of the room) but when she red going to the left to the bathroom her body went to the right. She said every time she tried to move left she could only go right and ended up against the wall. I was able to get her back to her bed and called for the nurse, who had left her alone in the room, and explained to her what happened. The nurse said why didn't you push the call button for help when you couldn't get to the bathroom by yourself. I told the nurse by that time she was too far away from the call button. Amber said she had yelled for help but no one came. (No one could hear her as she wasn't as loud as she thought she was). The nurse hadn't realized that this sort of thing could happen with a 17 year old girl who seemed to be doing so much better (she was in a regular hospital room). Amber was not left alone in her room again. She seemed to be doing very well but then things like that would happen.

She received a maintenance IVIG treatment (4 hour infusion) on August 23, 2011. She has not had any more IVIG treatments since then. She continues to take her seizure medicine her thyroid medicine. She goes to her endocrinologist every 6, but gets her blood drawn every 3 - 6 months to check her thyroid levels. She goes to her neurologist more often. At first she saw the neurologist every 2 weeks, then once a month, then every 2 months. Her neurologist is in charge of her IVIG treatments. Now Amber only needs to see neurologist every 3 to6 months depending on her symptoms.

Even though she doesn't have to get regular IVIG treatments any more, she still has some symptoms at times. Because her symptoms are not occurring often, her neurologist is just recording them to keep track of how she is doing. He doesn't seem to worry too much about symptoms happening ever so often, as long as the symptoms are not extremely severe and/or happening more frequently as he has to determine what could be permanent brain damage or actual symptoms of her disease becoming active again.

Her symptoms that happen on occasion are: headaches lasting for more than 5 hours, word finding difficulties, out of body experience (she feels that she is out of her body looking down at it), brain fog (had to concentrate, feeling fuzzy in the head), short term memory issues (she uses tools to help with that - such as setting an alarm to take her medicines and wring things down that she needs to remember), and being excessively tired. I believe Amber is extremely lucky as it took less than 2 weeks to come up with her diagnosis. The principal diagnosis is Hashimoto's Encephalopathy, and her secondary diagnosis is Hashimoto's Thyroiditis. It is my understanding that the longer it takes to diagnose this condition, the more damage that is done by the antibodies attacking one's own brain, which can result in lasting problems for the patient.

With very hard work on part, Amber was able to graduate high school on time. She will be attending beauty school to become nail technician. We are all hoping for the best for her to get through the beauty college and her state board exam to be licensed. Her doing this will tell us how much HE has affected her brain.

My daughter being diagnosed with this has been a life change experience, however, I am very grateful that she is still with us today and able to live her life. I hope she has a long and happy life. This I pray for her, my beautiful baby girl, Amber Rae.

Update November 2013:

Amber's headaches/migraines now happen about 20 days out of the month. Her neurologist is working with her to reduce the amount of headaches she is having. She has memory loss still. She does not remember a lot of things that had happened so she takes a lot of pictures for reminders of things happening in her life. She continues to get fatigued but she has accomplished quite a lot. She has now graduated beauty school (which she got 100% on her final exam) and she has also passed both parts of her State Board exam and is a licensed nail technician. While she was attending beauty school she also held down part time job which she still works at today and is also working at a local salon as a nail technician.

I am so very proud of my baby girl. She has been through so much and is not letting that get her down. She continues to live her life and just learns ways to make life easier as she goes (ex. she has alarms set for taking medicines, she takes notes/reminders for things she needs to remember).

I am so very grateful for all the doctors, nurses and staff at Toledo Children's Hospital (especially the PICU staff) for all the care they gave my daughter and for them being able to diagnose her illness as quickly as they did.

I would also like to thank Anji for starting the Hashimoto's Encephalopathy page on Facebook. My husband found the page, showed it to me, and it has been my lifeline since. Thanks to Anji, I have found several people with the same disease as my daughter and have learned a lot from them. They are definitely my new friends and I try to give back to them the best that I can.

I am also thankful for my Pastor coming and spending so much time with me at the hospital in the PICU. She was a great help as my family was in my time of need.

Amber was diagnosed at the age of 17, 2 1/2 months before her 18th birthday, and the summer beginning her senior year of high school. She is now 20 years old and living her life. A mother could not be prouder of her daughter than I am of Amber Rae.

IV. Loved Ones Speak Out

A Husband Shares: "My Hero"

My Name is Chad Fesler, husband to Anji Fesler. I wanted to provide a unique perspective of how one can overcome all the obstacles that one will face with HE. My wife Anji was diagnosed with HE back in December 0f 2004, this was after watching her deteriorate right before my eyes over 3 months prior of being in the hospital. I watched my wife lose the ability to talk, walk, feed herself, loss of memory, could not remember names, people, dates, numbers, etc. Once she was released from the hospital it was a slow process to recovery. Anji was at home but she was not comfortable in her own house and had lost her motherly instincts, to care for our child Zakk, who was only 1 at the time.

Slowly but surely memories came back to her and she began using her brain more and more. She started showing the emotions again that made Anji who she is: compassionate, loving, caring, happy, etc. She began to love our animals again, began loving and caring for our child, and had the determination and drive to get better.

Anji refused to give up on life and refused to be handicapped by this disease. She tried her best to start cooking again but bless her heart she couldn't follow instructions and would get confused at measurements, but she never gave up. She would see it through to the end. We as a family can now laugh at her pecan pies that were like soup and her mashed potatoes that were lumpy and inedible. Anji did not have a sense of balance and did not have or could not gauge and sense perspective in front of her. When she walked, her gate was awkward and clumsy. She would go to the grocery store and bang the shopping cart around every corner and aisle. She would go to the mall pushing Zakk in the stroller and would run into every shopper within five feet of her.

But through it all she refused to stop trying, refused to give up, and just persevered through making her body and mind work. After a few months, I made the decision to allow Anji to start driving again, against the mother-in-laws wishes. She started at first only driving in the neighborhood, to the gas station or grocery store that was within one mile of the house. She had her share of trial and errors driving along with way. Many times she would hit curbs, run over curbs, and hit the garage. After 6 months she began to grow confident in her ability to drive, communicate, care for the family, all daily routine activities. But now came the challenge of going back to work.

In June of 2005 Anji started back to her career as a social worker in the local school district. Like everything else Anji faced, there were daily if not hourly struggles that she faced: remembering people's names, communication with coworkers and students' families, staying organized, staying focused, etc. But before long, days turned into months and months turned into years. Anji continued to progress and get better because she pushed herself to do so. She had the inner will to live her life as she did before this disease impacted her life.

Anji is an inspiration to me and is the strongest person I have ever met. As I write this in November of 2013, if you met Anji you would never know that she had this debilitating disease. Anji actively works out, which I personally think assisted in bringing her back and is critical to helping the brain recover.

Anji works full time still as a social worker and receives exceptional reviews yearly. She is a wonderful wife, mother, friend, keeps this family together and moving forward. Yes there are still issues we deal with daily. From time to time there are issues with word finding, remembering names. She has nerve issues in her feet, legs, and has lost some sensitivity in some areas.

Anji still has issues with forgetfulness and has issues with numbers and dates. But with all these challenges Anji perseveres through it all, never complains of what cards she was dealt. One more thing through all of this: Anji lost hearing in one of her ears and partial loss in the other, and had to have both hips replaced, due to the long term exposure to steroids during her recovery. For those struggling with this disease who are frustrated with their disabilities, know there is hope. Know that for some of you, it can get better. The question is how bad and how hard do you want to work?

Through Love, strength and determination, Anji proved all others wrong and refused to become a victim and be told she could not accomplish or do something.

She is my hero, my strength, my friend....

Anji, I Love you for who you are!

A Parent Shares: "One Family's Story"

I have an adult family member who has Hashimoto's encephalopathy but it's not just the patient who is affected. This disease has widespread effects. Our loved one has had a total change in personality. Once a loving caring member of the family, they are now totally self-centered. Our family suffers emotionally, physically and financially from this illness. Those in the home are most affected but it reaches far into the extended family too. Most of the family hates being around the patient.

Our experiences started back in 2009. The patient was visiting with a friend and when they returned home, exhaustion had set in. After a few days of rest it didn't get any better. Then depression started. It was soon impossible for him/her to function; tears would flow for no reason. I was beginning to see changes but had no idea what lay ahead. We headed for our family doctor who agreed that something was wrong but wasn't sure what. After a few drugs for depression that didn't help a whole lot; the tests started. First a few simple tests. Results showed thyroid function was slightly off. They started Synthroid in the hopes that would help everything, but patient was still on a slow decline. Next came brain x-rays to see if the pituitary was the source of the problem. The results were enough to startle the radiologist. The pituitary was fine, but the radiologist was surprised the patient was still at home. He had no idea what was going on, he had never seen anything like this.

So off we went to a famous university hospital where we got the news that there was nothing wrong. This was a lifelong condition that was not the cause of any of the problems and the things we were facing were only the result of the depression. That was a diagnosis no one agreed with so on to more tests.

The next round of tests was blood work again but this time the doctor tested for antibodies. There was enough of an elevation to send us to a rheumatologist. Again confirmation that something was wrong but no idea what it could be. At least this doctor was concerned. After a few visits he was aware that the patient was getting worse. The patient was showing a lot of confusion. It was almost like living with an Alzheimer's patient: no idea as to what was real, time had lost all meaning, things that happened 15 years earlier were thought of as present. The doctor kept telling me if things get worse to go to the emergency room immediately but when I would call to report increase of mental confusion I would keep getting the same answer "if things get worse go to ER." I never did get any idea as to what kind of worse I needed to be concerned with.

This doctor finally was able to get us to a neurologist who cared. Once the neurologist saw the patient he had a few ideas. More tests, lots more tests. The patient continued to decline, confusion was now constant, as was the lethargy and depression, and again I was told "If things get worse go to the ER". It seemed like forever before we started to get some answers, but in reality it was less than 2 months. Finally, patient was admitted to the hospital for the last few tests and then finally a diagnosis and treatment.

Once on treatment the patient finally started to respond. But it was s-l-o-w. One of the hardest things I went through was that the patient forgot about the family members who had passes away years earlier. I relived the deaths many times before the patient ever grasped the fact that these people were gone.

I hate HE and the damage it has done to my family. I continue to love the patient but at the same time I hate the person they have become.

I know I have much to be thankful for, many patients went years without diagnosis, as ours came fairly quickly, and many suffer with pain. But still the changes are difficult to live with. I would love to have my former family member back again, and fear for the future if the patient out lives me. I can't imagine them being able to care for themselves or pursue medical care that is needed.

A Husband Shares: "A Roller Coaster Ride"

Being a caregiver for someone with Hashimoto's encephalopathy can be very difficult and confusing. It left me with a lot of emotions that were difficult to deal with, and hard to talk about. I'm sharing them in case you end up with some of these feelings, so you know you're not alone.

My wife had been having a lot of health problems, but the first sign to me that something was really wrong was when she came home one day shaking pretty hard, more like convulsions than anything else. At the time I thought she had pushed herself too hard, which was something she did now and then. It took me quite a while to learn that kind of shaking was called myoclonus, a not-uncommon side effect of quite a few ailments.

As her mental faculties degraded, other strange things began to occur. She began to lose self-awareness, and a lot of things around her no longer registered. There was a bit I could vividly remember where we crossed the street, and I actually had to pull her out of the way of oncoming traffic. If I hadn't, she would've been run over, but threats to herself of any sort didn't register at all. Social awareness also disappeared, and she couldn't pick up what anyone around her was thinking or feeling, especially me. At times she seemed really insensitive, and it was only later that I grasped that it wasn't any spitefulness, her brain wasn't picking up body language or noticing the dog asking to be let out. Her moods darkened, and there were large personality swings all over the shop, on days that she showed any emotion at all. It felt like she was no longer the person I married, and it was a very lonely time.

It's hard to describe the feelings I went through as my wife's illness progressed and lingered on further, months upon months onward. Looking back at it, I really wish I could've done more, but hindsight is 20/20, and at the time I did the best I could. Coming from a very healthy family, I had never encountered major illness and as time went on it was hard not to be annoyed. My upbringing was always sort of 'just put a BandAid on it, you'll be fine'. I was concerned, but as it progressed longer and longer it caused a very deep rift that was hard to get over - a pervasive resentment of why she couldn't just be better, or just get up and move along even if it was bad. At the same time stress was beginning to build; I had moved up to the United States only a few months prior, starting a new life, a new job, marriage. Tasks that used to be shared became on my shoulders alone, the domestic life began to crumble at the edges, and the resentment built some more.

It makes me feel bad to think on it, but suddenly I had another person to look after, all the duties now on me alone, and I had no energy left over from work to even pursue avenues to go down. I shudder to think about those with children or double work loads - that stress would be a killer. It was also hard not to react to it as if it was a character problem or a mental health issue, always with a negative connotation. 'What is wrong with her? She's broken.' people would think, with such a small amount of empathy. I would be dishonest if I also didn't mention that those thoughts crossed though my mind as well. It broke my heart when she just hugged me one day, breaking down with sobs, and the only thing she could say is 'I don't want to be a burden anymore'. People always assume that a mental illness means something is fundamentally flawed with the person. Some of the doctors even said it was just in her head! As if she would just pick to act that sick for the sake of it.

The further on it went though, the resentment gave way to helplessness. What could I do? She would sit there at home all day until I got back, either asleep or staring at the wall, not even having the brainpower to get bored! There was nothing, and doctor after doctor just come back with different ideas (everything from a bad migraine to West Nile Virus), but no decision and no plan to get her better. She was offloaded from specialist to specialist, each one brilliant in his field, but no one put it all together. In the end, we went through 27 doctors before finding one who figured it out and treated her.

There are quite a few issues that happen with Hashimoto's Encephalopathy, and I think the reason why it gets misdiagnosed all the time is the sheer amount of symptom overlap that it has with other 'less exotic' conditions. If I knew back then what I do now, I would've pushed the doctors to try treatment for Hashimoto's Encephalopathy. The solution was so simple it was anticlimactic: a short dose of steroids with a maintenance dose after that, and now she's back. Not always to what she was before, but so much better that I cannot describe it properly.

A Daughter Shares: "HE Mom"

I never lived with a mother with HE: I lived with Energizer Bunny mom. My mom could work, clean and play circles around me when I was in my twenties and she in her late 40's. We would take business trips together. I would be in bed hours before she would even return to the room. In the morning she was always the first one up and out the door. I saw my mother nap once in my whole life. I remember being so worried because she had to be really, really sick if she was napping. She barely ever sat down! She could work a 50 hour week in a fast paced retail environment, have a spotless house, laundry caught up and a homemade meal for her family of 6 (and anyone else who showed up) effortlessly.

That mom is gone. She has been replaced with HE mom. Don't get me wrong HE mom is still ultra caring, fun loving and optimistic (and somehow her house is still clean!) but things have changed. She gets tired and confused. It takes several attempts to stand up out of a chair....she actually sits now! It is scary to watch your vibrant mom slow down.

Mom's mom had terrible thyroid issues. So it was not a surprise when mom was diagnosed with thyroid. But HE is hard to detect and mom had several other autoimmune diseases that all presented at around the same time. Weird "things" started to happen that, at the time, you wouldn't even consider a symptom of anything. She was embarrassed by the color of her hands. Dry skin? She would forget words. Stress over her sick mother? She would get a funny feeling she couldn't describe while driving. Panic attack? I think it was when she started to lose her balance and nearly lost control of her bowels that she took matters into her own hands. Mom will tell you, you have to be your own advocate. You know your body. You know what is normal and what is not. Do not let a doctor tell you nothing is wrong when you know something is. Seek another opinion. And another. And another.

Let's face it, no one has heard of HE unless they know someone who has it. So when mom was diagnosed it didn't mean a lot to us kids. After all, we are all grown and out of the house and didn't really see the symptoms. So it stayed sort of abstract in our minds. Even when the doctor told her she would have to quit her job it wasn't really real to me yet. And then something happened. Something so huge, it could not be ignored. Mom listened to the doctor and she quit her job! Something was definitely wrong with my mom. Her job defined her. She worked her way up from a part time sales associate when we were just kids, to a manager, to a store owner. She thrived in her stores. She loved helping someone find just the right thing to make them feel wonderful, or the perfect gift for a loved one. She worked! It was what she did.

This lone act of quitting made me nervous. I researched...a little, because there is not enough known about HE to research a lot. It is not good news when researching HE. It is scary and depressing and my mom has it! And I am here, 8 hours away!

So what can we, grown children of HE moms do? We can be patient. Mom may move slower. She may talk funnier. She may rest more often. Trust she is much more frustrated over this than you are. We can listen. HE mom is going to get frustrated. She is going to get depressed. She is going to need someone to listen to her and remind her that behind HE is still that amazing, loving, happy go lucky mother who loves to help others. We can get google ready. We are going to have a lot of medical jargon flung at us! Most, most importantly we can take charge of our own health. Not enough is known about HE to be sure it is not hereditary. Tell your doctor your family medical history (and watch their reaction to the words Hashimoto Encephalopathy - if they even know what it is). Get your yearly physical and just be aware. Be aware of anything you just think is "off" and be your own advocate.

I still don't understand HE and I probably never will. But I understand I have a new mom. A mom who needs to rest. A mom who sleeps in. A mom who does not take a 3 mile walk every day. A mom who can't shop all day and cook all night. A mom who repeats herself. A mom who doesn't always get things right. A mom who jumbles words and can't always get across what she is saying. A mom who can't drive long distances. A mom who trips when nothing is there to trip over.

There is a blessing in all of this though. Mom has always said we learn from what we go through and we get to help others through it too. HE mom gets to bless many others with her knowledge of and experience with HE. Energizer Bunny mom is still going...just a little slower. And she is still working. She is working as an advocate for HE awareness. And that may be the most important job she has ever had.

A Friend Shares: "Different Country, Different Journey"

After the shock of our friend's HE onset settled, my next thought was thank God she is still with us and whatever is going on we will walk through it at her side.

I kept thinking of the old story about comparing a major life change to having bought a ticket to one country and ending up someplace else. We didn't expect our brilliant friend to ever be facing these challenges. But, she is still with us and showing improvement and is still loved and respected. It's just a different country, and different journey.

We have experienced her speech difficulties, the memory lapses. We have witnessed the tremors and unsteady gait. And we have stayed calm and moved forward.

Yes, the friendship is different. But all friendships change over the years. Ours had a major shift applied to it. The friendship was strong to start with and can weather any blow that HE wants to toss our way. Life doesn't give anyone any guarantees.

The person we loved years ago is still there. She just needs a little more patience sometimes and a little more understanding. That's what friends do. We can long for what used to be, it's the human way. But it is much more rewarding to find the joy that is still there. It is going to take more than HE to take her away from the people who love her.

A Daughter Shares: "Silver Lining"

The heartache caused by watching a loved one struck down by any illness is an indescribable pain. The fear and anxiety caused by an unknown illness stealing the person you once knew cannot possibly be explained.

Watching helplessly as the mental decline that should happen over a lifetime overtakes your loved one in a matter of hours…to be told there is no answer and that it is most likely mental illness causes a new anguish.

Going to specialists who seem to refuse to help for fear of being thought foolish by their colleagues who are skeptical of HE, and all the while the person you are fighting for is withering in front of your eyes and there is nothing you can do.

You learn the limitations of your loved one and begin a new relationship with this different person. You quietly mourn the loss of their former self and dare not imagine how they must feel to be a shadow of themselves.

To dwell on this causes an ocean of sadness to engulf you, so instead you choose to embrace this new version. You choose to be thankful your loved one is still here and is strong enough to begin anew.

I have never been more proud of my mother than I have been watching the grace and dignity she has shown in her battle. She is an inspiration and a blessing, and I am thankful for her every day. There are many silver linings that have come with her illness and they are my focus. Her life is different now, but she has embraced the changes and adopted unanticipated roles, developing and devoting herself to new passions.

My hope is that the medical community as a whole will become informed and take action to improve the lives of those who are suffering from HE.

A Mother Shares: "The Daughter Is Teaching the Mother"

How has Hashimoto's Encephalopathy affected my life? It has forever changed it, even though I'm not the one afflicted with this horrid disease. Rather, my daughter contracted this disease approximately eight years ago.

As parents we try to protect our children, no matter their age. This disease has left me feeling so helpless against trying to protect my daughter and although I may feel helpless, HE will not leave me feeling hopeless!

I have seen this disease change my daughter's life drastically. It has caused her to have so many major struggles just to get through the day. It has robbed her of many of the mother/daughter memories we have shared together. If I could I would take this disease on myself, if it would free her from it.

As you read my little excerpt in this wonderful book, you may be surprised by what I'm about to say next. Believe it or not something good has come out of this awful, life changing event in my daughter's life. HE has enabled me to discover what a courageous and brave daughter I have. I always knew how wonderful she was...but now she is also my heroine! Instead of letting this disease take her life from her, I have seen her use it to make this a better world for others who share this disease with her.

Not a day goes by that my heart doesn't break over what my daughter has to deal with, however I'm grateful it has enabled me to see her courageous heart.

Others could learn from her how to react to adversity in one's life... I know I have. The daughter is teaching the mother.

A Friend Shares: "Longing for What Has Been Taken"

My best friend has Hashimoto's Encephalopathy. We used to live about a block from each other, our children growing up together, and our social lives intertwined. We were both intelligent women who dropped out of college and finally, together, found the courage to go back, got our degrees, and then pursued graduate school. A few years ago, I moved across the country to take a job but we remained close through the wonders of communication technology and airplanes. We had a number of 2-3 day vacation visits, sometimes with a husband in tow, and always thoroughly enjoying each other's presence and company.

In retrospect, our last "normal" visit was an incredible gift of time we gave each other. We had 4 full days in 2011 to do nothing but be with each other. No husbands, no children, no responsibilities. Our last visit, it turns out, was the last time we had ordinary conversations about our lives bereft of health issues or concerns.

A few weeks after our last normal visit, I noticed a post on Facebook about my friend having some medical emergency at work and ending up in the hospital. I called the hospital and they put me through to my friend. She said she was tired, but otherwise seemed ok. Her speech with me had normal volume, rate, and rhythm. She thought she may have had a stroke at work because she suddenly couldn't speak but the neurologist thought she had a complex migraine. It seemed like she just had something weird occur and the medical folk were checking to see what it could have been. She reported no loss of movement or anything else abnormal except for a continuing headache.

However, within a week, her ability to speak disintegrated. She emailed that she thought she had another stroke because she was having a horrible time speaking about anything but concrete subjects. She also wrote, "Thank God for the written word, and the computer. If I didn't have my laptop I would feel completely trapped inside my head. With the laptop, I can write words down and express myself. I have to do a lot of editing, but at least I can communicate. I just realized that when I try to talk about intangibles, I am composing and spitting out the words one by one as though typing, but without the keyboard. Does that make sense? The process is almost identical. Interesting!!!! That's why it doesn't flow. Because I have to think about each word individually, the same as if typing."

Then things got really bad for her and she asked to be left alone. She was trying to get a diagnosis but her health and cognitive functions were diminishing. She was hospitalized and learned she had been having seizures during the past week and was hopeful her doctor would have some treatment that would give her relief and stabilize her condition. Her days consisted of 3-4 hours of being awake, naps on and off throughout the day, and 12-hours of sleep at night.

I returned to visit her a couple of months later and found her nearly unable to speak a full sentence without severe breaks between syllables and floundering for words. This was so uncharacteristic of my friend, who was a word wizard and grammarian who would correct the children's school's newsletters and return them with the errors noted in red ink.

In addition, she could not remember more than one step at a time. For example, making bacon and eggs for breakfast was too many steps! At this time, she also required multiple naps each day for her tiredness and to keep seizures at bay. It was a very distressing visit for me because my dearest friend was so physically weak and unable to communicate more than short difficult-to-assemble sentences.

Because of her speech issues, email or Facebook became the only way to communicate because it gave her time to think of what she wanted to say, write it, correct it, and then post it or send it. She told me it was like she had all these files in her head, but had no idea which file had the word in it that she wanted. She continued to pursue specialists hoping to get a definitive diagnosis, but none occurred. Around this time, she realized she had such profound memory loss, she would not be able to return to her career, and reluctantly retired.

Finally, she was going to the Mayo clinic. But that turned out to be unhelpful because the specialist she needed to see wasn't there during her visit. She was depressed afterward because, in spite of abnormal test results, they suggested her problems were better addressed by a psychiatrist!

Her memory continued to decline and although we remained in contact, she would forget to update me about important things and would forget I had sent emails. I noticed a baby shower photo on Facebook and asked her about it. She realized she had forgotten to tell me her daughter was having a baby – in about a month!

I visited her shortly after her granddaughter was born. She was better able to speak but it was still a lot of work for her and her speech had abnormal rhythm. She was also now using a wheelchair because of concerns about falling, as well as fatigue.

A few months later, however, she found a new doctor and was hopeful for the future. She seemed through her emails and posts to be doing much better. She was spending time with her new little granddaughter, too, and that seemed to help her focus. Then, when the baby was a few months old, she moved to be closer to her daughter and the baby, and was well enough to spend a lot of time with her granddaughter.

When I visited recently, she seemed more normal than at any of my earlier visits. Her speech was clearer and faster, although it still had odd rhythms. However, in the midst of a conversation, she suddenly went limp and became mentally non-responsive. She had strange oscillations of her trunk along with vomiting and reciting gibberish. This went on for over an hour. Her husband said they now know to just let it run its course because she will be ok. And that is what happened. A few hours later, we talked and she had absolutely no memory of our earlier meeting and conversation.

I hate this disease. It has robbed us of the comfortable friendship and intimacy we had nurtured over decades, forcing us to reinvent our communication. And, as for me, I long for the days of easy conversations and making and recalling memories on the fly.

A Son Shares: "The Person Within"

Every time I got a call that there had been another episode, my greatest fear was that this was the time I would no longer recognize my mother. She had explained to me that Hashimoto's Encephalopathy took the file cabinet of her brain and dumped out all of her files and put them back in a new, seemingly random order. I would collect myself and get on a train headed home, hoping that she would still have the ability to find her files.

The most memorable of her hospital stays was in the final year of my undergraduate studies at The School of the Art Institute of Chicago. The workload was almost unbearable, sometimes leaving time for sleep only every third night. It was during this time that my mother was hospitalized in Chicago. I would finish my 7 hour studio course downtown and jump on the south bound pink line train to the hospital, armed with the vegan dinners that she requested to balance out the standard hospital food (I'm not sure I've ever seen someone so thrilled to see a kale salad).

Every night was a confirmation that she was still there. This woman, who sometimes could not speak, only look at me with tears welling from frustration with her inability to string together words, was still my mother. I would spend a couple of hours with her and head back to the studio to work, usually through the night, and repeat.

This all happened far too soon after she finished her law degree (and as Valedictorian, I might add, when she was 50 years old), while she was in the midst of a highly successful career at a major, national law firm.

When HE began to take hold she was forced to stop working. Her work as an attorney was truly a passion, and as time passed it became clear that the chance for her to continue the pursuit of this passion was fading. It wasn't fair, but it was not over. She needed to see that even if she never went back to work it was not over. She showed me what it was to have an unrivaled love and passion for one's work, and I would show her what that meant to me.

The fear of losing the person my mother once was has subsided. She is not the person she once was; she has grown and changed in the most beautiful ways. Her passion has not faded, but shifted. She has dedicated her time to helping those struggling to understand HE, and continues to inspire me with her commitment to the marginalized. Every day is a new struggle, and with every treatment comes a new hope. In times of great struggle and great disappointment we see truth within a person. The journey of understanding HE is one that has provided me with great insight into the core of my mother. As she continues to adapt and grow I see that she is not only the woman that I have always loved admired, but a better version of this person.

V. Resources

While the patient stories paint a vivid picture of life with HE, and the struggle to find a diagnosis and appropriate treatment, for those who want more we provide the following resources which will allow readers to delve as deeply into HE as they wish.

In this section you will find citations to the majority of scientific articles about HE published between 2010 and 2013, including internet addresses for finding them online.

The second section of this chapter lists online groups and communities of HE patients and websites that offer additional information.

The final section lists organizations that you may wish to contact and/or support.

Scientific Articles and Case Studies

Articles Published in 2013

Hashimoto's Encephalopathy Presenting Periodic Synchronous Discharge, as a Differential Diagnosis for Creutzfeldt-Jakob Disease.till

T Muramatsu, T Hamano, N Shirafuji, A Matsunaga, M Ikawa, and M Yoneda.

Clinical Neurology, 2013 Oct 4; 53 (9): 716-720.

doi: 10.5692/clinicalneurol.53.716

Abstract:

http://www.ncbi.nlm.nih.gov/pubmed/24097320

Hashimoto's Encephalopathy: four cases and review of literature.

Gülen Gul Mert, Ozden Ozgur Horoz, M. Ozlem Herguner, Faruk Incecik, R. Dincer Yildizdas, Neslihan Onenli Mungan, Bilgin Yuksel, and Sakir Altunbasak.

International Journal of Neuroscience, 2013 Oct 2.

doi: 10.3109/00207454.2013.836706

Abstract:

http://informahealthcare.com/doi/abs
/10.3109/00207454.2013.836706

Clinical and Neuropathological Findings in Hashimoto's Encephalopathy: a case report.

Daniele Imperiale, Carmelo Labate, Roberto Testi, Alessandra Romito, and Stefano Taraglio.

Neurological Sciences, 2013 Sep 24. [Epub ahead of print]

doi: 10.1007/s10072-013-1554-y

Extract:

http://link.springer.com/article/10.1007%2Fs10072-013-1554-y#page-1

Clinical Manifestations and Treatment Response of Steroid in Pediatric Hashimoto Encephalopathy.

Hee Joon Yu, Jeehun Lee, Dae Won Seo, and Munhyang Lee.

Journal of Child Neurology, 2013 Sep 20. [Epub ahead of print]

doi: 10.1177/0883073813499823

Abstract:

http://jcn.sagepub.com/content/early/2013/09/19/0883073813499823.abstract

Subacute Cognitive Deterioration with High Serum Anti-Thyroid Peroxidase Antibodies: two cases and a plea for pragmatism.

Kurt Segers Philippe Braconnier, Francis Corazza, Luisa Divano, Asmaa Mabrouk, Jean Robberecht, and Murielle Surquin.

Psychogeriatrics, 2013 Sep 17; 13 (3): 175-179.

doi: 10.1111/psyg.12018

Abstract:

http://onlinelibrary.wiley.com/doi/10.1111/psyg.12018/abstract

A Case of Hashimoto's Encephalopathy Misdiagnosed as Viral Encephalitis.

Lei He, Mei Li, Xiao-Hong Long, Xiang-Pen Li, and Ying Peng.

American Journal of Case Reports, 2013 Sep 13; 14: 366-369.

doi: 10.12659/AJCR.889312

Full Text:

http://www.ncbi.nlm.nih.gov/pmc/articles/PMC3775618/

Anti-NMDAR Encephalitis Misdiagnosed as Hashimoto's Encephalopathy.

M Mirabelli-Badenier, R Biancheri, G Morana, S Fornarino, L Siri, ME Celle, E Veneselli, A Vincent, R Gaggero, and MM Mancardi.

European Journal of Paediatric Neurology, 2013 Aug 19. [Epub ahead of print]

doi: 10.1016/j.ejpn.2013.07.002

Abstract:

http://www.ncbi.nlm.nih.gov/pubmed/23953644

Diagnostic and Therapeutic Aspects of Hashimoto's Encephalopathy.

Inan Olmez, Harold Moses, Subramaniam Sriram, Howard Kirshner, Andre H Lagrange, and Siddharama Pawate.

Journal of the Neurological Sciences, 2013 Aug 15; 331 (1-2): 67-71. [Epub 2013 Jun 5]

doi: 10.1016/j.jns.2013.05.009

Abstract:

http://www.ncbi.nlm.nih.gov/pubmed/23759502

Immune Dysregulation and Autoimmunity in Bipolar Disorder: synthesis of the evidence and its clinical application.
Sanil Rege and Suzanne J Hodgkinson.
Australian & New Zealand Journal of Psychiatry,
2013 Aug 1. [Epub ahead of print]
doi: 10.1177/0004867413499077
Abstract:
http://anp.sagepub.com/content/early/2013/08/19/0004867413499077.abstract

Adult-Onset Temporal Lobe Epilepsy, Cognitive Decline, Multi-Antiepileptic Drug Hypersensitivity, and Hashimoto's Encephalopathy: two case studies.
Ofer Sadan, Estelle Seyman, Elissa L Ash,
Svetlana Kipervasser, and Miri Y Neufeld.
Epilepsy & Behavior Case Reports, 2013 Aug; 1: 132-135.
doi: 10.1016/j.ebcr.2013.07.004
Full Text:
http://www.sciencedirect.com/science/article/pii/S2213323213000352

Recurrent Status Epilepticus Associated with Hashimoto's Encephalopathy.

H Visée, C Mabiglia, V Vanderaspoilden, MD Gazagnes, and G Glibert.

Epilepsy & Behavior Case Reports, 2013 Aug; 1: 113-117.

doi: 10.1016/j.ebcr.2013.06.003

Full Text:

http://www.sciencedirect.com/science/article/pii/S2213323213000297

Spectroscopic Correlation and Role of Azathioprine in Long-Term Remission in Patients of Hashimoto Encephalopathy.

Harpreet Singh, Sucharita Ray, Shalini Agarwal, Raj Pal Verma, Paulomi Talapatra, and Vikas Gupta.

Annals of Indian Academy of Neurology, 2013 Jul; 16 (3): 443-446.

doi: 10.4103/0972-2327.116936

Full Text:

http://www.ncbi.nlm.nih.gov/pmc/articles/PMC3788305/

Paediatric Autoimmune Encephalopathies: clinical features, laboratory investigations and outcomes in patients with or without antibodies to known central nervous system autoantigens.

Yael Hacohen, Sukhvir Wright, Patrick Waters, Shakti Agrawal, Lucinda Carr, Helen Cross, Carlos De Sousa, Catherine DeVile, Penny Fallon, Rajat Gupta, Tammy Hedderly, Elaine Hughes, Tim Kerr, Karine Lascelles, Jean-Pierre Lin, Sunny Philip, Keith Pohl, Prab Prabahkar, Martin Smith, Ruth Williams, Antonia Clarke, Cheryl Hemingway, Evangeline Wassmer, Angela Vincent, and Ming J Lim.

Journal of Neurology, Neurosurgery & Psychiatry, 2013 Jul; 84 (7): 748-755. [Epub 2012 Nov 22]

doi:10.1136/jnnp-2012-303807

Full Text:

- http://jnnp.bmj.com/content/early/2012/11/21/jnnp-2012-303807.full

Hashimoto's Encephalopathy Masquerading as Chronic Meningitis – case of a middle-aged female with review of literature.

Akhila Kumar Panda, Gopinath G, Siddharth Maheswari, Vachan Jayant Mehta, and Lomesh Bhirud.

Indian Journal of Medical Specialities, 2013 Jun 2.

doi: 10.7713/ijms.2013.0021

Full Text:

http://www.ijms.in/articles/5/1/hashimoto%E2%80%99s-encephalopathy-masquerading.html

The Biomarker and Treatment in Hashimoto's Encephalopathy.

T Kishitani, A Matsunaga, and M Yoneda.

Japanese Journal of Clinical Medicine, 2013 Jun; 71 (5): 893-897.

Abstract:

http://europepmc.org/abstract/MED/23777101

Improvement of Cerebral Hypoperfusion with Levothyroxine Therapy in Hashimoto's Encephalopathy Demonstrated by 99mTc-HMPAO-SPECT.

WJ Schnedl, S Mirzaei, SJ Wallner-Liebmann, E Tafeit, H Mangge, R Krause, and RW Lipp.

European Thyroid Journal, 2013 Jun; 2: 116-119.

doi: 10.1159/000348523

Abstract:

http://www.karger.com/Article/Abstract/348523

Hashimoto's Encephalopathy in the Intensive Care Unit.

B Chaigne, E Mercier, D Garot, A Legras, PF Dequin, and D Perrotin.

Neurocritical Care, 2013 Jun; 18 (3): 386-390.

doi: 10.1007/s12028-013-9834-1

Extract:

http://link.springer.com/article/10.1007/s12028-013-9834-1#page-1

Steroid-Responsive Thalamic Lesions Accompanying Microbleeds in a Case of Hashimoto's Encephalopathy with Autoantibodies Against α-enolase.

Yoshitaka Yamaguchi, Manabu Wada, Haruko Tanji, Katsuro Kurokawa, Toru Kawanami, Kazuyo Tanji, Makoto Yoneda, and Takeo Kato.

Internal Medicine, 2013 Jun; 52 (11): 1249-1253.

doi: 10.2169/internalmedicine.52.9373

Full Text:

https://www.jstage.jst.go.jp/article/internalmedicine/52/11/52_52.9373/_pdf

A Patient with Hashimoto's Encephalopathy Presenting with Convulsive Seizure Alone as the Initial Symptom.

Atsushi Mizuma, Yoshiaki Goto, Wacoh Takahashi, Shunya Takizawa, and Shigeharu Takagi.

Clinical Medicine Insights: Case Reports, 2013 May 5; 6: 75-77.

doi: 10.4137/CCRep.S10390

Full Text:

http://www.ncbi.nlm.nih.gov/pmc/articles/PMC3656644/

Hashimoto's Encephalopathy.

Neelkanth Bapat, Vinayak Hingane, and Pavan Hanchnale.

Journal, Indian Academy of Clinical

Medicine, 2013 May; 14 (1): 71-72.

Full Text:

http://medind.nic.in/jac/t13/i1/jact13i1p71.pdf

Immune-Mediated Pediatric Epilepsies.

Christian G Bien and Angela Vincent.

Handbook of Clinical Neurology, 2013 May; 111: 521-531.

doi: 10.1016/B978-0-444-52891-9.00055-5

Abstract:

http://www.sciencedirect.com/science/article/pii/B9780444528919000555

Hashimoto's Encephalopathy Presenting With Altered Mental Status and Myoclonus and Co-Occurring With Psoriasis.

Arshi Naz, Muhammad M Sheikh, and Mayada Issa.

Journal of Medical Cases, 2013 May; 4 (5): 300-303.

doi: 10.4021/jmc1144w

Full Text:

http://www.journalmc.org/index.php/JMC/article/view/1144/639

Hashimoto's Encephalopathy: identification and long-term outcome in children.

Nafissa Mamoudjy, Christian Korff, Hélène Maurey, Gaëlle Blanchard, Dominique Steshenko, Marie-Noëlle Loiseau-Corvez, Béatrice Husson, Raja Brauner, Marc Tardieu, and Kumaran Deiva.

European Journal of Paediatric Neurology, 2013 May; 17 (3): 280-287.

doi: 10.1016/j.ejpn.2012.11.003

Abstract:

http://www.sciencedirect.com/science/article/pii/S1090379812002346

Thyroid Autoantibodies in Pregnancy: their role, regulation and clinical relevance.

Francis S Balucan, Syed A Morshed, and Terry F Davies.

Journal of Thyroid Research, 2013 Apr 18; 2013: 182472.

doi: 10.1155/2013/182472

Full Text:

http://www.ncbi.nlm.nih.gov/pmc/articles/PMC3652173/

(Note: this article does not specifically deal with HE. However, it describes the effects of thyroid antibodies on pregnancy, making it highly relevant to HE patients who are or wish to become pregnant.)

Autoimmune Epilepsy as Drug-Resistant Epilepsy.
M Zare.
Iranian Journal of Neurology, 2013 Apr; 12 (1): 43.
Abstract:
http://ijnl.tums.ac.ir/index.php/ijnl/article/view/345

Brain Hypoperfusion on Tc-99m-Ethylene Dicysteine Diethyl Ester Single-Photon Emission Computed Tomography in Hashimoto's Encephalopathy.
María Luz Domínguez Grande, Ana Constantino, Juan Ignacio Rayo, Justo Serrano, Jose Rafael Infante, Lucia Garcia, and Carmen Duran.
Indian Journal of Nuclear Medicine,
2013 Apr; 28 (2): 102–104.
doi: 10.4103/0972-3919.118231
Full Text:
http://www.ncbi.nlm.nih.gov/pmc/articles/PMC3800302/

Hashimoto's Encephalopathy and Autoantibodies.

M Yoneda.

Brain and Nerve, 2013 Apr; 65 (4): 365-376.

Abstract:

http://www.ncbi.nlm.nih.gov/pubmed/23568984

Hashimoto's Encephalopathy: a rare cause of status epilepticus.

A Doe De Maindreville, C Gombert, A Thiriaux, M Chaunu, and S Bakchine.

Revue Neurologique, 2013 Apr; 169 (4): 345-349. [Epub 2013 Feb 26]

doi: 10.1016/j.neurol.2012.10.014

Abstract:

http://www.ncbi.nlm.nih.gov/pubmed/23452828

Serial Changes in Diffusion-Weighted Magnetic Resonance Images with Hypoperfusion on Brain SPECT in a Case of Hashimoto's Encephalopathy: understanding pathophysiology of Hashimoto's encephalopathy.

Sung Jae Kim, Eun Hwan Jeung, Mi Kyung Park, Sunseob Choi, and Kyung Won Park.

Dementia and Neurocognitive Disorders, 2013 Mar 31; 12 (1): 29-32.

doi: 10.12779/dnd.2013.12.1.29

Full Text:

http://synapse.koreamed.org/search.php?where=aview&id=10.12779/dnd.2013.12.1.29&code=0196DND&vmode=FULL

Hashimoto's Encephalopathy Presenting as Acute Cognitive Decline in an Elderly Male.

Madan Raj Aryal, Smith Giri, Naba Raj Mainali, and Karen Smith.

World Journal of Neurology, 2013 Mar 28; 3 (1): 1-3.

doi: 10.5316/wjn.v3.i1.1

Full Text:

http://www.wjgnet.com/2218-6212/full/v3/i1/1.htm

Limbic Encephalitis Associated With Elevated Antithyroid Antibodies.

Yael Hacohen, Sonia Joseph, Rachel Kneen, Paul Eunson, Jean-Pierre Lin, Angela Vincent, and Ming Lim.

Journal of Child Neurology, 2013 Mar 20. [Epub ahead of print]

doi: 10.1177/0883073813480392

Abstract:

http://jcn.sagepub.com/content/early/2013/03/19/0883073813480392.abstract

Epilepsy Associated with Systemic Autoimmune Disorders.

Orrin Devinsky, Adam Schein, and Souhel Najjar.

Epilepsy Currents, 2013 Mar; 13 (2): 62-68.

doi: 10.5698/1535-7597-13.2.62

Full Text:

http://epilepsycurrents.org/doi/full/10.5698/1535-7597-13.2.62

Acute Psychiatric Presentation of Steroid-Responsive Encephalopathy: the under recognized side of autoimmune thyroiditis.

Cristiano Carlone, Liliana Todini, Isabella Marini, Michele Majorana, Sara Casciato, Anna Teresa Giallonardo, Mauro Pallagrosi, Massimo Salviati, and Massimo Biondi.

Rivista di Psichiatria, 2013 Mar; 48 (2): 169-173.

doi: 10.1708/1272.14042

Full Text:

http://www.rivistadipsichiatria.it/articoli.php?archivio=yes&vol_id=1272&id=14042

Hashimoto's Encephalopathy with Hippocampus Involvement Detected on Continuous Arterial Spin Labeling.

Makoto Ishitobi, Makoto Yoneda, Masamichi Ikawa, Akiko Matsunaga, Kanji Ueno, Hirohiko Kimura, and Yuji Wada.

- Psychiatry and Clinical Neurosciences, 2013 Feb 25; 67 (2): 128-129.
- doi: 10.1111/pcn.12019
- Abstract:
- http://onlinelibrary.wiley.com/doi/10.1111/pcn.12019/abstract

Hashimoto's Encephalopathy Associated with Anti-NAE Autoantibodies: analysis of 101 patients.

Akiko Matsunaga, Toru Kishitani, Tomoko Muramatsu, Tomomi Kame, Masamichi Ikawa, Yasunari Nakamoto, and Makoto Yoneda.

Neurology, 2013 Feb 12; 80 (Meeting Abstracts 1): S29.002.

Abstract:

http://www.neurology.org/cgi/content/meeting_abstract/80/1_MeetingAbstracts/S29.002

Cognitive Impairments in Hashimoto's Encephalopathy: a case-control study.

Jianhong Wang, Jun Zhang, Lan Xu, Yunbo Shi, Xunyi Wu, and Qihao Guo.

PLOS ONE, 2013 Feb 8; 8 (2): e55758.

doi:10.1371/journal.pone.0055758

Full Text:

http://www.plosone.org/article/info:doi/10.1371/journal.pone.0055758

Hashimoto's Encephalopathy as a Treatable Adult-Onset Cerebellar Ataxia Mimicking Spinocerebellar Degeneration.

A Matsunaga, M Ikawa, A Fujii, Y Nakamoto,
M Kuriyama, and M Yoneda.
European Neurology, 2013 Feb; 69 (1): 14-20.
doi: 10.1159/000342217
Abstract:
http://www.ncbi.nlm.nih.gov/pubmed/23128836

A Diagnosis Sometimes Overlooked?

Louis Björkman and Dan Gustafsson.
Acta Pædiatrica, 2013 Jan; 102 (1): 92. [Epub 2012 Dec 11]
doi: 10.1111/apa.12042
Full Text:
http://onlinelibrary.wiley.com/doi/10.1111/apa.12042/full

Hashimoto Encephalopathy Presenting as Progressive Myoclonus Epilepsy Syndrome.

Ravindra Arya, Vidhu Anand, and Maya Chansoria.
European Journal of Paediatric Neurology, 2013
Jan; 17 (1): 102-104. [Epub 2012 Jul 25]
doi: 10.1016/j.ejpn.2012.07.001
Full Text:
http://www.ejpn-journal.com/article/
S1090-3798(12)A00149-3/fulltext

Articles Published in 2012

Nonconvulsive Status Epilepticus as the First Manifestation of Hashimoto's Encephalopathy.

JG Lee, DW Shin, JY Seo, KB Lee, IM Jang, H Roh, and MY Ahn.

Journal of Korean Epilepsy Society, 2012 Dec; 16 (2): 63-66.

Abstract:

http://www.koreamed.org/SearchBasic.php?RID=1103JKES/2012.16.2.63&DT=1

Hashimoto's Encephalopathy: a case report.

lkay Keleş, Gizem Güneş, and Ahmet Tiryaki.

Bulletin of Clinical Psychopharmacology, 2012 Dec; 22 (1): S117.

Abstract:

http://www.psikofarmakoloji.org/pdf/22_11_115.pdf

Hashimoto Encephalopathy: a rare intricate syndrome.

Juraj Payer, Tomas Petrovic, Lubomir Lisy, and Pavel Langer.

International Journal of Endocrinology & Metabolism, 2012 Dec; 10 (2): 506-514.

doi: 10.5812/ijem.4174

Full Text:

http://endometabol.com/?page=article&article_id=4174

Hashimoto's Encephalopathy as the Cause of Deteriorating Consciousness During Treatment of Leptomeningeal Carcinomatosis from Breast Cancer.

Yi-Hsin Liang, Pei-Fang Wu, Ching-Hung Lin, and Yen-Shen Lu.

Journal Clinical Oncology, 2012 Nov 20; 2012: e358-e359. [Epub 2012 Oct 8]

doi: 10.1200/JCO.2012.44.0826

Full Text:

http://jco.ascopubs.org/content/early/2012/10/03/JCO.2012.44.0826.full.pdf

Autoimmune Encephalitis in Children.

Thais Armangue, Mar Petit-Pedrol, and Josep Dalmau.

Journal of Child Neurology, 2012 Nov; 27 (11): 1460-1469. [Epub 2012 Aug 29]

doi: 10.1177/0883073812448838

Full Text:

http://jcn.sagepub.com/content/27/11/1460.long

Opsoclonus as a Manifestation of Hashimoto's Encephalopathy.

R Salazar, C Mehta, N Zaher, and D Miller.

Journal of Clinical Neuroscience, 2012 Oct;
19 (10) 1465-1466. [Epub 2012 Aug 11]
doi: 10.1016/j.jocn.2012.02.012

Abstract:
http://www.ncbi.nlm.nih.gov/pubmed/22889978

A Patient with Steroid Responsive Encephalopathy Associated with Autoimmune Thyroiditis.

Benjamin K Tsang, Nicholas Crump, and Andrew J Hughes.

Journal of Clinical Neuroscience, 2012 Oct;
19 (10): 1459-1460. [Epub 2012 Aug 9].
doi: 10.1016/j.jocn.2012.02.014

Abstract:
http://www.jocn-journal.com/article/S0967-5868(12)00146-4/abstract

A Selective Memory Deficit Caused by Autoimmune Encephalopathy Associated with Hashimoto Thyroiditis.

C Koros, A Economou, G Mastorakos, A Bonakis, N Kalfakis, and SG Papageorgiou.

Cognitive and Behavioral Neurology, 2012 Sep; 25 (3): 144-148.

doi: 10.1097/WNN.0b013e31826b7ed7

Abstract:

http://www.ncbi.nlm.nih.gov/pubmed/22960439

Hashimoto's Encephalopathy Cases: Chinese experience.

Yi Tang, Yi Xing, Michael T Lin, Jin Zhang, and Jianping Jia.

BMC Neurology, 2012 Jul 24; 12: 60.

doi:10.1186/1471-2377-12-60

Full Text:

http://www.biomedcentral.com/1471-2377/12/60

Hashimoto's Encephalopathy.

B Chaigne, E Beaufils, Y Jouan, J Magnant, F Maillot, T Constans, C Hommet, and K Mondon.

La Revue de Médecine Interne, 2012 Jul; 33 (7): 390-395. [Epub 2012 Apr 3]

doi: 10.1016/j.revmed.2012.02.009

Abstract:

http://www.ncbi.nlm.nih.gov/pubmed/22475954

Steroid-Responsive Encephalopathy Associated with Hashimoto Thyroiditis.

Petra Zimmermann and Enno Stranzinger.

Pediatric Radiology, 2012 Jul; 42 (7): 891-893. [Epub 2011 Dec 30]

doi: 10.1007/s00247-011-2309-7

Extract:

http://link.springer.com/article/10.1007%2Fs00247-011-2309-7#page-1

Hashimoto Encephalopathy and Peripheral Neuropathy in an Italian Adolescent.

V Salpietro, V Granata, A Polizzi, K Mankad, S Briuglia, R Gallizzi, G Tortorella, and M Ruggieri.

The Child Journal of Pediatrics, 2012 Jun; 1 (2): 9.

Full Text:

http://www.thechild.it/archives/2012/number2/page.php?id=9

Hashimoto's Encephalopathy: neuropsychological findings.

I. Mazzù, S Mosti, C Caltagirone, and GA Carlesimo.

Neurological Sciences, 2012 Jun; 33 (3): 653-356. [Epub 2011 Oct 13]

doi: 10.1007/s10072-011-0813-z

Extract:

http://link.springer.com/article/10.1007%2Fs10072-011-0813-z#page-1

Pearls & Oy-sters: Hashimoto encephalopathy.

Mitra Afshari, Zahra S Afshari, and Stephan U Schuele.

Neurology, 2012 May 29; 78 (22): e134-e137.

doi: 10.1212/WNL.0b013e3182582fd4

Full Text:

http://www.neurology.org/content/78/22/e134.full

Hashimoto's Encephalopathy.

Gouranga Santra, Dibyendu De, Sibaji Phaujdar, Aniruddha Rudra, and Partha Sarathi Dutta.

Journal of the Association of Physicians of India, 2012 May; 60: 48-50.

Full Text:

http://www.japi.org/may_2012/13_cr_hashimotos_encephalopathy.html

Steroid-Responsive Encephalopathy Associated with Graves' Disease.

R Dobrescu, D Morosanu, S Jercalau, C Tiu, and C Badiu.

Endocrine Abstracts (European Society of Endocrinology), 2012 May; 2012 (29): P1708.

Abstract:

http://www.endocrine-abstracts.org/ea/0029/ea0029p1708.htm

Autoimmune Encephalopathy Associated with Thyroid Autoantibodies as the Cause of Reversible Cognitive Impairment.
Natallia Maroz, Nechama Bernhardt, and Robert Dobbin Chow.
Journal of Community Hospital Internal Medicine Perspectives, 2012 Apr 30; 2 (1): 11453.
doi: 10.3402/jchimp.v2i1.11453
Full Text:
http://www.jchimp.net/index.php/jchimp/article/view/11453/html

Rituximab Therapy in a Patient with Recurrent Hashimoto's Encephalitis (HE), and Progressive Encephalomyelitis with Rigidity and Myoclonus (PERM).
Darine Kassar, Srikanth Damodaram, Stanley Iyadurai, and Pratap Chand.
Neurology, 2012 Apr 25; 78 (Meeting Abstracts 1): P04.164.
doi: 10.1212/WNL.78.1_MeetingAbstracts.P04.164
Abstract:
http://www.neurology.org/cgi/content/meeting_abstract/78/1_MeetingAbstracts/P04.164

Immunopathology of Autoantibody-Associated Encephalitides: clues for pathogenesis.

Christian G Bien, Angela Vincent, Michael H Barnett, Albert J Becker, Ingmar Blümcke, Francesc Graus, Kurt A Jellinger, David E Reuss, Teresa Ribalta, Jürgen Schlegel, Ian Sutton, Hans Lassmann, and Jan Bauer.

Brain, 2012 Apr 25; 135 (5): 1622-1638.

doi:10.1093/brain/aws082

Full Text:

http://brain.oxfordjournals.org/content/135/5/1622.full

Steroid-Responsive Encephalopathy Associated with Autoimmune Thyroiditis Presenting as Confusion, Dysphasia, and Myoclonus.

Stephen A Ryan, Claire Kennedy, and Hugh J Harrington.

Case Reports in Medicine, 2012 Apr 17; 2012: 782127.

doi: 10.1155/2012/782127

Full Text:

http://www.hindawi.com/journals/crim/2012/782127/

Hashimoto's Encephalopathy Presenting with Micrographia as a Typical Feature of Parkinsonism.

K Inoue, J Kitamura, M Yoneda, E Imamura, and H Tokinobu.

Neurological Sciences, 2012 Apr; 33 (2): 395-397.

doi: 10.1007/s10072-011-0750-x

Extract:

http://link.springer.com/article/10.1007%2Fs10072-011-0750-x#page-1

A Case of Hashimoto's Encephalopathy Presenting with Seizures and Psychosis.

Min-Joo Lee, Hae-Sang Lee, Jin-Soon Hwang, and Da-Eun Jung.

Korean Journal of Pediatrics, 2012 Mar; 55 (3): 111-113.

doi: 10.3345/kjp.2012.55.3.111

Full Text:

http://www.ncbi.nlm.nih.gov/pmc/articles/PMC3315621/?tool=pubmed

Paroxysmal Kinesigenic Dyskinesia as the Initial Symptom of Hashimoto Encephalopathy.

Ming-Yuan Liu, She-Qing Zhang, Yong Hao, and Hui-Min Zheng.

CNS Neuroscience & Therapeutics, 2012 Mar; 18 (3): 271-273.

doi: 10.1111/j.1755-5949.2012.00297.x

Abstract:

http://onlinelibrary.wiley.com/doi/10.1111/j.1755-5949.2012.00297.x/abstract

Hashimoto's Encephalopathy Presenting with Multiple Cranial Nerve Palsies and Hemiparesis: a case report.

Santanu Saha, Riddhi Das Gupta, Adreesh Mukherjee, Arijit Singha, Dhiman Das, and Mrinal Kanti Roy.

International Journal of Case Reports and Images, 2012 Mar; 3 (5): 31-35.

doi:10.5348/ijcri-2012-05-122-CR-7

Full Text:

http://www.ijcasereportsandimages.com/archive/2012/005-2012-ijcri/007-05-2012-saha/ijcri-00705201277-saha-full-text.php

Anti-Thyroid Antibodies in Two Patients with Subacute Dementia, Ataxia, and Myoclonus.

Daniel Kondziella, Klaus Hansen, Teresa Gonzalez, Peter Gideon, Ingelise Christiansen, and Finn Sellebjerg.

Ugeskrift for Læger, 2012 Feb 27; 174 (9): 577-579. [full text in Danish; summary in English]

Full Text:

- http://www.ugeskriftet.dk/videnskab/antithyroideaantistof-hos-patienter-med-subakut-dementiel-udvikling-ataksi-og-myoklonus

Hashimoto Encephalopathy Causing Drug-Resistant Status Epilepticus Treated with Plasmapheresis.

Ömer Bektas, Arzu Yılmaz, Tanil Kendirli, Zeynep Sıklar, and Gülhis Deda.

Pediatric Neurology, 2012 Feb; 46 (2): 132-135.

doi: 10.1016/j.pediatrneurol.2011.11.009

Abstract:

http://www.ncbi.nlm.nih.gov/pubmed/22264710

Steroid-Responsive Encephalopathy Subsequently Associated with Alzheimer's Disease Pathology: a case series.

Farrah J Mateen, Keith A Josephs, Joseph E Parisi, Daniel A Drubach, Richard J Caselli, Kejal Kantarci, Clifford Jack, and Bradley F Boeve.

Neurocase, 2012 Feb; 18 (1): 1-12. [Epub 2011 Jun 30]

doi: 10.1080/13554794.2010.547503

Full Text:

http://www.ncbi.nlm.nih.gov/pmc/articles/PMC3184345/

Articles Published in 2011

Hashimoto's Encephalopathy in Children and Adolescents.

Ilknur Erol, Semra Saygi, and Füsun Alehan.

Pediatric Neurology, 2011 Dec; 45 (6): 420-422.

doi:10.1016/j.pediatrneurol.2011.09.010

Abstract:

http://www.ncbi.nlm.nih.gov/pubmed/22115010

Recurrent Partial Seizures with Ictal Yawning as Atypical Presentation of Hashimoto's Encephalopathy (Steroid-Responsive Encephalopathy Associated with Autoimmune Thyroiditis).

S Casciato, C Di Bonaventura, L Lapenta, J Fattouch, G Ferrazzano, M Fanella, F. Di Fabio, M. Pasquini, MA Amendolea, M Manfredi, M Prencipe, and AT Giallonardo.

Epilepsy & Behavior, 2011 Dec; 22 (4): 799-803.

doi: 10.1016/j.yebeh.2011.09.023

Abstract:

http://www.sciencedirect.com/science/article/pii/S1525505011005567

Encephalopathy Associated with Autoimmune Thyroid Disease (Hashimoto's Thyroiditis) Presenting as Depression: a case report.

Chao-Yu Liu, Mei-Chih Meg Tseng, and Po-Hsien Lin.

General Hospital Psychiatry, 2011 Nov; 33 (6): 641.e7-641.e9.

doi:10.1016/j.genhosppsych.2011.05.019

Abstract:

http://www.ncbi.nlm.nih.gov/pubmed/21762998

Infectious Disease or Hashimoto's Encephalopathy Flares: a case report.

Wenyan Huang, Chang Xia, and Marie Chatham.

Seizure, 2011 Nov; 20 (9): 717-719.

Full Text:

http://www.seizure-journal.com/article/S1059-1311(11)00131-2/fulltext

Hashimoto's Encephalopathy: systematic review of the literature and an additional case.

Narriane Chaves P de Holanda, Denise Dantas de Lima, Taciana Borges Cavalcanti, Cynthia Salgado Lucena, and Francisco Bandeira.

The Journal of Neuropsychiatry & Clinical Neurosciences, 2011 Sep 1; 23 (4): 384-390.

doi:10.1176/appi.neuropsych.23.4.384

Full Text:

http://neuro.psychiatryonline.org/article.aspx?articleID=181292

Central Nervous System Vasculitis with Positive Antithyroid Antibodies in an Adolescent Boy.

Sarah L Tsai, Evan C Lewis, Erick Sell, and Sharon Whiting.

Pediatric Neurology, 2011 Sep; 45 (3): 189-192.

doi: 10.1016/j.pediatrneurol.2011.04.012

Abstract:

http://www.ncbi.nlm.nih.gov/pubmed/21824569

Spontaneous Remission of Encephalopathy Associated with Autoimmune Thyroid Disease in a Patient with Graves' Disease: a rare occurrence in a rare clinical picture.

Yagoub Elfaki, Donal O'Shea, and Gianluca Tamagno.

International Journal of Endocrinology & Metabolism, 2011 Sep; 9 (4): 373-376.

doi: 10.5812/Kowsar.1726913X.3183

Full Text:

http://endometabol.com/?page=article&article_id=3183

Non-Convulsive Status Epilepticus of Frontal Origin as the First Manifestation of Hashimoto's Encephalopathy.

G Monti, M Pugnaghi, A Ariatti, L Mirandola, G Giovannini, S Scacchetti, P Nichelli, and S Meletti.

Epileptic Disorders, 2011 Sep; 13 (3): 253-258.

doi: 10.1684/epd.2011.0457

Abstract:

http://www.ncbi.nlm.nih.gov/pubmed/21896425

Steroid-Responsive Encephalopathy and Autoimmune Thyroiditis in a Young Boy.

Sanket D Shah and Hema Murali.

Pediatric Neurology, 2011 Aug; 45 (2): 132-134.

doi:10.1016/j.pediatrneurol.2011.04.002

Abstract:

http://www.ncbi.nlm.nih.gov/pubmed/21763957

Steroid-Responsive Hashimoto Encephalopathy Mimicking Creutzfeldt-Jakob Disease.
Domenico Santoro, Irene Colombo, Isabella Ghione, Lorenzo Peverelli, Nereo Bresolin, Monica Sciacco, and Alessandro Prelle.
Neurological Sciences, 2011 Aug; 32 (4): 719-722. [Epub 2011 May 10]
doi: 10.1007/s10072-011-0610-8
Extract:
http://link.springer.com/article/10.1007%2Fs10072-011-0610-8#page-1

Steroid-Responsive Encephalopathy in Autoimmune Thyroiditis: clinical spectrum and MRI observations in three cases.
K Dinkar, Sanjib Sinha, AB Taly, PS Bindu, and RD Bharath.
Annals of Indian Academy of Neurology, 2011 Jul; 14 (3): 205-207.
doi: 10.4103/0972-2327.85897
Full Text:
http://www.annalsofian.org/article.asp?issn=0972-2327;year=2011;volume=14;issue=3;spage=205;epage=207;aulast=Dinkar

Why the Confusion in Hashimoto's Encephalopathy?
Bodiabaduge AP Jayasekera, Michael Anthony McShane, Prem Roy, and Geetha Anand.
BMJ Case Reports, 2011 Jun 16; 2011: bcr0320114020.
doi: 10.1136/bcr.03.2011.4020
Full Text:
http://www.ncbi.nlm.nih.gov/pmc/articles/PMC3118897/

A Methodology for Assessing Treatment Response in Hashimoto's Encephalopathy: a case study demonstrating repeated computerized neuropsychological testing.
Brian L Brooks and Karen M Barlow.
Journal of Child Neurology, 2011 Jun; 26 (6): 786-791. [Epub 2011 Feb 10]
doi: 10.1177/0883073810391532
Abstract:
http://jcn.sagepub.com/content/26/6/786.abstract

Progressive Impairment of Cognition and Motor Function: Hashimoto encephalopathy.
Peter Tzakas and Sze Wan Sit.
Canadian Medical Association Journal,
2011 May 17; 183 (8): E495-E497.
doi: 10.1503/cmaj.100007
Full Text:
http://www.ncbi.nlm.nih.gov/pmc/articles/PMC3091936/

Hashimoto's Encephalopathy: a long-lasting remission induced by intravenous immunoglobulins.
Jelena Drulović, Sladjana Andrejević, Branka Bonaci-Nikolić, and Vesna Mijailović.
Vojnosanitetski Pregled, 2011 May; 68 (5): 452-454.
doi: 10.2298/vsp1105452d
Full Text:
http://www.doiserbia.nb.rs/img/doi/0042-8450/2011/0042-84501105452D.pdf

A Case of Hashimoto Encephalopathy: clinical manifestation, imaging, pathology, treatment, and prognosis.

Weiqin Zhao, Jimei Li, Jiawei Wang, Yanjun Guo, Houzhen Tuo, Zhimin Kang, Bin Jiang, Rui Wang, and Dexin Wang.

The Neurologist, 2011 May; 17 (3): 141-143.

doi: 10.1097/NRL.0b013e3182173341

Abstract:

http://www.ncbi.nlm.nih.gov/pubmed/21532381

Tremor and Myoclonus Heralding Hashimoto's Encephalopathy.

K Gücüyener, A Serdaroğlu, A Bideci, Y Yazman, A Ş Soysal, and P Cinaz.

Journal of Pediatric Endocrinology and Metabolism, 2011 Apr; 13 (8), 1137-1142.

doi: 10.1515/JPEM.2000.13.8.1137

Extract:

http://www.degruyter.com/view/j/jpem.2000.13.8/jpem.2000.13.8.1137/jpem.2000.13.8.1137.xml

Hashimoto's Encephalopathy in the Setting of Subclinical Hypothyroidism.
Vasile M Bota and Dominic F Corrigan.
International Journal of Case Reports and Images, 2011 Apr; 2 (4): 19-22.
doi:10.5348/ijcri-2011-04-30-CR-5
Full Text:
http://www.ijcasereportsandimages.com/archive/2011/004-2011-ijcri/005-04-2011-bota/ijcri-00504201155-bota-full-text.php

Presenile Dementia: a case of Hashimoto's encephalopathy.
CSY Chong, JLM Leung, IHH Wong, PW Ng, and MYK Miao.
East Asian Archives of Psychiatry, 2011 Mar; 21 (1): 32-36.
Full Text:
http://easap.asia/journal_file/1101_V21N1_p32.pdf

Steroid Responsive Encephalopathy Associated with Autoimmune Thyroiditis (SREAT) or Hashimoto's Encephalopathy: a case and review.

Susan W Lee, Stacy Donlon, and Jason P Caplan.

Psychosomatics, 2011 Mar; 52 (2): 99-108.

doi: 10.1016/j.psym.2010.12.010

Abstract:

http://www.ncbi.nlm.nih.gov/pubmed/21397101

Manic Symptoms Associated with Hashimoto's Encephalopathy: response to corticosteroid treatment.

Shuai-Ting Lin, Cheng-Sheng Chen, Pinchen Yang, and Cheng-Chung Chen.

The Journal of Neuropsychiatry and Clinical Neurosciences, 2011 Feb 1; 23 (1): E20-E21.

doi: 10.1176/appi.neuropsych.23.1.e20

Full Text:

http://neuro.psychiatryonline.org/article.aspx?articleid=179748

Hashimoto's Encephalopathy.

Joana Ramalho and Mauricio Castillo.

Radiology Case Reports, 2011 Jan 31; 6 (1): 445.

doi: 10.2484/rcr.v6i1.445

Full Text:

http://radiology.casereports.net/index.php/rcr/article/viewArticle/445/793

Time for the Endocrinologists to Expand Their Awareness of and Contribution to the Diagnosis and Management of Encephalopathy Associated with Autoimmune Thyroid Disease.

Gianluca Tamagno and Gadintshware Gaoatswe.

Hormones, 2011 Jan; 10 (1): 36-38.

Full Text:

http://www.hormones.gr/pdf/HORMONES%202011-36-38.pdf

Articles Published in 2010

Successful Response to Intravenous Immunoglobulin as Rescue Therapy in a Patient with Hashimoto's Encephalopathy.

Rodrigo Cornejo, Pablo Venegas, Daniela Goñi, Alvaro Salas, and Carlos Romero.

BMJ Case Reports, 2010 Dec 29.

doi: 10.1136/bcr.09.2010.3332

Full Text:

http://www.ncbi.nlm.nih.gov/pmc/articles/PMC3027904/

Paediatric Hashimoto Encephalopathy, Refractory Epilepsy and Immunoglobulin Treatment – unusual case report and review of the literature.

I Berger, Y Castiel, and T Dor.

Acta Pædiatrica, 2010 Dec; 99 (12): 1903-1905. [Epub 29 Oct 2010]

doi: 10.1111/j.1651-2227.2010.01967.x

Abstract:

http://www.ncbi.nlm.nih.gov/pubmed/20678162

A Series Report of Autoimmune Hypothyroidism Associated with Hashimoto's Encephalopathy: an under diagnosed clinical entity with good prognosis.

Hemanta Kumar Nayak, Mrudul Kumar Daga, Rakshit Kumar, Sandeep Kumar Garg, Naresh Kumar, and Pankaj Kumar Mohanty.

BMJ Case Reports, 2010 Nov 23; 2010: bcr0120102630.

doi: 10.1136/bcr.01.2010.2630

Full Text:

http://www.ncbi.nlm.nih.gov/pmc/articles/PMC3027635/

Hashimoto Encephalopathy: clinical and MRI improvement following high-dose corticosteroid therapy.

Thashi Chang, MTM Riffsy, and Padma S Gunaratne.

The Neurologist, 2010 Nov; 16 (6): 394-396.

doi: 10.1097/NRL.0b013e3181d6b6f6

Abstract:

http://www.ncbi.nlm.nih.gov/pubmed/21150392

Hashimoto's Encephalopathy Presenting with Neurocognitive Symptoms: a case report.

Carlos Canelo-Aybar, David Loja-Oropeza, Jose Cuadra-Urteaga, and Franco Romani-Romani.

Journal of Medical Case Reports, 2010 Oct 25; 4: 337.

doi:10.1186/1752-1947-4-337

Full Text:

http://www.jmedicalcasereports.com/content/4/1/337

Hashimoto Encephalopathy with Fulminant Myocarditis.

Mark Podberezin, Matthew N Meriggioli, Alberto Locante, Andras Voros, Tibor Valyi-Nagy, and André Kajdacsy-Balla.

Pathology - Research and Practice, 2010 Oct 15; 206 (10): 720-722. [Epub 2010 May 21]

doi: 10.1016/j.prp.2010.02.015

Abstract:

http://www.ncbi.nlm.nih.gov/pubmed/20494527

Autoimmune Dementia: clinical course and predictors of immunotherapy response.
Eoin P.Flanagan, Andrew McKeon, Vanda A Leonnon, Bradley F Boeve, Max R Trenerry, K Meng Tan, Daniel A Drubach, Keith A Josephs, Jeffrey W Britton, Jayawant N Mandrekar, Val Lowe, Joseph E Parisi, and Sean J Pittock.
Mayo Clinic Proceedings, 2010 Oct; 85 (10): 881-897.
doi: 10.4065/mcp.2010.0326
Full Text:
http://www.ncbi.nlm.nih.gov/pmc/articles/PMC2947960/

Electrophysiological Tests in a Case of Hashimoto's Encephalopathy.
S Shibayama, A Igaki, M Kuroda, M Honnda, S Fujii, Y Wada, K Inuzumi, M Takeda, and M Koshiba.
Rinsho Byori, 2010 Oct; 58 (10): 986-989.
Abstract:
http://www.ncbi.nlm.nih.gov/pubmed/21077288

Steroid Responsive Encephalopathy Associated with Autoimmune Thyroiditis Presenting with Late Onset Depression.

FA Babtain.

Neurosciences (Riyadh), 2010 Jul; 15 (3): 196-199.

Abstract:

http://www.ncbi.nlm.nih.gov/pubmed/20831030

Clinical Reasoning: a 9-year-old girl with seizures and encephalopathy.

Thy P Nguyen and Lisa M El-Hakam.

Neurology, 2010 Jun 1; 74 (22): e97-e100.

doi: 10.1212/WNL.0b013e3181e0f75e

Full Text:

http://www.neurology.org/content/74/22/e97.full

Steroid-Responsive Myeloneuropathy Associated with Antithyroid Antibodies.

Recai Turkoglu and Erdem Tuzun.

The Journal of Spinal Cord Medicine, 2010 Jun; 33 (3): 278-280.

Full Text:

http://www.ncbi.nlm.nih.gov/pmc/articles/PMC2920124/

Encephalopathy Associated with Autoimmune Thyroid Disease in Patients with Graves' Disease: clinical manifestations, follow-up, and outcomes.
Gianluca Tamagno, Yahya Celik, Rafael Simó, Marcel Dihné, Kazumi Kimura, Giorgio Gelosa, Byung I Lee, Caroline Hommet, and Giovanni Murialdo.
BMC Neurology, 2010 Apr 28; 10: 27.
doi:10.1186/1471-2377-10-27
Full Text:
http://www.biomedcentral.com/1471-2377/10/27

Steroid Responsive Encephalopathy in Cerebral Amyloid Angiopathy: a case report and review of evidence for immunosuppressive treatment.
Raoul P Kloppenborg, Edo Richard, Marieke ES Sprengers, Dirk Troost, Piet Eikelenboom, and Paul J Nederkoorn.
Journal of Neuroinflammation, 2010 Mar 9; 7: 18.
doi:10.1186/1742-2094-7-18
Full Text:
http://www.jneuroinflammation.com/content/7/1/18

Hashimoto Encephalopathy in a Preschool Girl.

Manuel Castro-Gago, Carmen Gómez-Lado, Mercedes Maneiro-Freire, Jesús Eirís-Puñal, and Manuel Bravo-Mata.

Pediatric Neurology, 2010 Feb; 42 (2): 143-146.

doi:10.1016/j.pediatrneurol.2009.09.011

Abstract:

http://www.ncbi.nlm.nih.gov/pubmed/20117754

Clinical Manifestations, Diagnostic Criteria and Therapy of Hashimoto's Encephalopathy: report of two cases.

Milija Mijajlovic, Mihailo Mirkovic, Jelena Dackovic, Jasna Zidverc-Trajkovic, and Nadezda Sternic.

Journal of the Neurological Sciences, 2010 Jan 15; 288 (1): 194-196. [Epub 2009 Oct 28]

doi:10.1016/j.jns.2009.09.030

Abstract:

http://www.ncbi.nlm.nih.gov/pubmed/19846119

Undetected Hashimoto Encephalopathy – a diagnostic challenge in child psychiatry and child neurology.
Renate Voll.
Zeitschrift für Kinder- und Jugendpsychiatrie und Psychotherapie, 2010 Jan; 38 (1): 21-27.
doi: 10.1024/1422-4917.a000003
Abstract:
http://www.ncbi.nlm.nih.gov/pubmed/20047173

Note: The list above contains content currently available to the public online. Additional content access may be available via libraries or educational institutions.

A list of additional, earlier articles about Hashimoto's Encephalopathy appears at: http://henotebook.wordpress.com/case-studies/

Support Groups

Facebook Communities and Pages:

"Hashimoto's Encephalopathy (HE) / Autoimmune Encephalopathy"

https://www.facebook.com/groups/251477975360/

A group devoted solely to Hashimoto's Encephalopathy patients and caregivers; also a good resource for those who believe they might have HE and want to learn more.

* * *

"Encephalitis Global"

https://www.facebook.com/groups/2369586237/

A group for patients/survivors/caregivers of all types of encephalitis or encephalopathy, including HE

* * *

"For Those Diagnosed with Hashimoto's Encephalopathy/SREAT"

https://www.facebook.com/groups/346906815423323/

A group open ONLY to those who have received a medical diagnosis of Hashimoto's Encephalopathy, and for parents of children diagnosed with HE

* * *

"Autoimmune Encephalitis Alliance"
https://www.facebook.com/AEalliance

A resource page for information about autoimmune encephalitis in general – not specific to HE. It is the official Facebook page for the Autoimmune Encephalitis Alliance, a nonprofit organization.

* * *

"Children with Hashimoto's Encephalopathy"
https://www.facebook.com/ChildrenwithHE

A support group for parents of children with HE:

Non-Facebook web-based support group:
"Encephalitis Global"
http://www.inspire.com/groups/encephalitis-global/?ref=as&asat=44736407

An internet based support groups for patients and caregivers of all types of encephalitis and encephalopathy, including HE).

* * *

Email-based support group:

HELPS at Topica.com — to join, send an email to: HELPS-subscribe@topica.com

Organizations and Informational Websites

Hashimoto's Encephalopathy SREAT Alliance "HESA" www.hesaonline.org

HESA is a registered nonprofit organization formed in 2012, dedicated to shedding light on HE/SREAT by collecting, compiling and sharing information. HESA also raises funds to support scientific research. Its website provides information and links to a variety of resources for patients, physicians, caregivers, and others interested in this poorly understood disorder.

Autoimmune Encephalitis Alliance www.aealliance.org

The Autoimmune Encephalitis Alliance is a nonprofit started by families and patients affected by all forms of autoimmune encephalitis, including HE. It is based in Durham North Carolina.

Hashimoto's Encephalopathy Study (website) http://henotebook.wordpress.com/

This highly informative website was created by an electrical engineer with HE, and provides a wealth of information for patients and families, including easy to understand descriptions of various aspects of HE and treatment options, some with illustrations.

The Encephalitis Society

www.encephalitis.info/information/types-of-encephalitis/types-of-autoimmune-encephalitis/

This is a UK-based group dedicated to all forms of encephalitis, including autoimmune varieties.

NIH Office of Genetic and Rare Diseases Information Center – www.rarediseases.info.nih.gov/gard/8570/hashimotos-encephalitis/more-about-this-disease

This is the National Institutes of Health page which provides information about Hashimoto's Encephalopathy.

11801337R00276

Printed in Great Britain
by Amazon.co.uk, Ltd.,
Marston Gate.